THE
ONE STOP
KNEE
SHOP

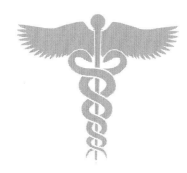

JACK E. JENSEN, M.D. FACSM

AOK Publishing Houston

AOK Publishing, Houston 77055
Copyright 2007 by Jack E. Jensen, M.D.
First edition published 2007
Printed in United States of America
09 08 07 06 05 04 03 02 01 00 10 9 8 7 6 5 4 3 2 1

Nothing can substitute for your physician's expertise. This book is not intended to replace common sense or a doctor's advice. Given the differences between patients, only your doctor can render a definitive medical diagnosis and recommend treatment for you and your family.

ISBN: 1-4196-5196-X
ISBN-13: 978-1419651960
Library of Congress Control Number : 2006909481

Visit www.booksurge.com to order additional copies.

Accolades for *The One Stop Knee Shop*

"Dr. Jack Jensen, eminently qualified and experienced orthopedic surgeon, has written the (now) defining book regarding knee health in a logical, common-sense and understandable style, covering injury-prevention and rehabilitation from injury and knee surgery. *The One Stop Knee Stop* provides a straight-forward blueprint for athletes of all abilities in recreational or competitive sports to maintain "healthy knees." I genuinely regret that I did not have the benefit of the information contained in *The One Stop Knee Shop* available during my personal competitive career."

Al Lawrence, 1956 and 1960 Olympian and Author of *The Self-Coached Runner* and *Running and Racing After 35*.

"Expertly written, *The One Stop Knee Shop* is the most complete and authoritative guide for knee care available. Dr. Jensen thoroughly educates the reader on how to best to maintain healthy knees and joints in the context of the whole person. He dedicates an entire chapter to arthritis, including clear explanations of conditions, symptoms, solutions, tips for improvement, how to cope, and directives on what every patient needs to know in regards to treatment options as well as keys to a healthy lifestyle. Not only is this book an excellent reference for patients, it is also a smart read for physicians, who stand to gain a wealth of knowledge from this practical and easy-to-understand presentation on the knee."

William Fleming, M.D., President, Harris County Medical Society and Speaker of the House of Delegates of the Texas Medical Association.

"Dr. Jensen is a real person. He is on the sidelines of most Houston high school games and college games in order to lend his help if needed. I know him to be a really interesting person who just happens to be an expert in the field of operating and helping patients recover from injuries. I can't tell you how many young and sometimes old athletes he has helped. He has also helped *prevent* many injuries by teaching.

Preventative medicine is one thing, but preventing surgery is another and Dr. Jack Jensen is *the* best in that area...."

Craig Roberts, Sports Director, Houston KPRC TV, KTBU TV, KIOL FM.

"Dr. Jensen's passion towards his specialty clearly shines through in this book. *The One Stop Knee Shop* clearly explains how the knee works with the rest of the body, which preventative measures to take against damage, how to understand a diagnosis, as well as treatment for and recuperation from a variety of specific problems. With this book, Dr. Jensen empowers patients with the information they need to take control of their situation, manage the relationship with their physician, and make a complete recovery. I recommend that all my gymnasts read this book!"

Bela Karolyi, World-Renowned USA Gymnastics Coach

"In all my years of reading books by doctors I have never come across one that is so forthright and so informative to all levels, whether lay person or medical practioner. Dr. Jensen captures all the facets of the knee and puts them in an order that is very reader friendly. He has something here that other authors have never been able to communicate to all people. It is very well done and I will recommend this book to all my players."

Bill Norris, Association of Tennis Professionals Sports Medicine Committee, ATP World Tour

"I have always said that the knees are the vital link between a person and the ground. Keeping them healthy is of utmost importance for being able to exercise at any level. Dr. Jensen's information will help you to both keep your knees in working order and to also pinpoint problems if you have them."

Mark Allen, 6 Time Ironman Triathlon World Champion

"This book is not only for injured persons, but is an essential read for athletes, exercisers, and anyone else looking to prevent injury. Dr. Jensen provides easy to follow, invaluable advice on protecting your knees from injury and rehabilitating them to full capacity if you have already suffered a knee crisis."

Herschel Walker, All-American Football Player, Heisman Trophy Winner, University of Georgia Athlete of the Century.

"Dr. Jensen impressively articulates a holistic approach to knee health, addressing general exercise and diet recommendations in additional to surgical and alternative medicinal options. Unlike other volumes on the subject of knees, this book explains in detail the effect nutrition can have on the musculoskeletal system, and offers sound, scientifically-proven nutritional and physical fitness information so that you can live a healthy, active life free from injury and free from pain."

Catherine Kruppa, MS, RD, LD – Licensed Dietitian and Member of "Dr. Phil's Empowerment Team."

"The One Stop Knee Shop is well written and quite approachable, despite the technical nature of its topic. The author does a fine job of explaining medical concepts and human anatomy in a light-hearted, conversational manner that is neither condescending nor intimidating, and still delivers accurate and informative details. Furthermore, the book offers a considerable amount of good advice for maintaining the health of one's knees, and best of all, is not just aimed at athletes or weekend warriors."

Ellen T. Marsh, *New York Times* **Best-Selling Author**

About the Author

Jack E. Jensen, M.D., F.A.C.S.M., is a board-certified orthopedic surgeon and medical director of the Athletic Orthopedics and Knee Center, an integrated health care plaza specializing in the care of knees. After performing as a collegiate athlete, Dr. Jensen attended medical school at The University of Kansas. He completed his orthopedic surgery residency at the University of Texas, and then went on to receive further training with some of the leading pioneers in the field at the University of Oregon, where he completed a surgical fellowship in Sports Medicine. Dr. Jensen, who has been distinguished with the title Fellow of the American College of Sports Medicine, has worked his sports medicine wares at the Goodwill Games, the World Championships of Gymnastics, the U.S. Olympic Training Center, and the Olympic Games. He has also served as orthopedic consultant to the United States Gymnastic Federation, team physician to Karolyi's Gymnastics, the USA Swimming Foundation, the Association of Tennis Professionals, and as orthopedic physician to numerous Olympic and professional athletes. Additionally, Dr. Jensen has worked with the Houston Rockets, the Houston Astros, The Houston Oilers, the Houston Texans, Cirque du Soleil, Houston Wranglers Tennis, The US Clay Court Tournament, The Masters Cup, and has served as Team Physician for the Missouri Tigers. Dr. Jensen, a recreational athlete who hikes, bikes, hunts, scuba dives, plays tennis, plays golf, swims, and runs marathons, is a member of the American Orthopedic Society for Sports Medicine, a member of the U.S. Olympic Sports Medicine Society, and a Fellow of the American Academy of Sports Physicians. A former associate editor of Medicine and Science in Sports and Exercise, he has co-authored numerous scientific articles in peer-reviewed publications, as well as a book for athletes and gymnasts, *A Healthy 10!*

Contents

Preface

When I first thought about titling this book, I wanted to call it *The Miracle Knee.* That's because in spite of two decades as an orthopedic surgeon specializing in athletic knee injuries, I have not gotten over my wonder of the knee. Little more than miscellaneous bones, ligaments, and cartilage held together in what seems an improbable assembly, the knee is capable of fantastic feats of speed, power, and grace.

Understanding my appreciation for the knee explains in part why I wrote this book, but understanding what led me to focus my medical practice on knees in the first place will explain more. Several events in the development of orthopedics happened to coincide with milestones in my life that made orthopedics in general and athletic knee injuries in particular a natural for my life's calling.

Another reason is that when I co-wrote *A Healthy 10!,* which was published in 1992, I intended it for use with all kinds of athletes, not just gymnasts. Patients need resources to turn to after they leave the doctor's office because it is easy for them to get overloaded when they are undergoing examination and evaluating options for therapy. If they have an injured knee, simply negotiating a visit to an orthopedist can be a struggle. *A Healthy 10!* is helpful because it offers a glimpse of my approach to a winning athletic lifestyle, which includes safe training, supportive nutrition, tips on fulfilling potential, and a brief review of the major musculoskeletal groups in the body and typical injuries.

In contrast, *The One Stop Knee Shop* focuses on just one aspect of the musculoskeletal system and gives readers the kind of in-depth explanations that they could never get in a book overview of the entire body. Injuries, in particular, have a way of getting a person's attention, especially if they impede walking. Such immobility fosters an interest in learning how to regain knee health and maintain it. Serving all patients with that interest is my intent in writing this book.

Having been on both sides of the stethoscope also explains my commitment to better communication between doctor and patient.

As a high school athlete, I played football and basketball and ran track; in college, I was a varsity letterman. As a lifelong recreational athlete, I ski, run, bike, play golf, swim, scuba dive, hike, hunt—you name it. The only serious knee injury I suffered during my years in athletic competition was sustained not on the field but on the road in a car wreck. This brought knees to my attention from the patient's point of view. Also early in my athletic career, I assisted other hurt athletes, and I discovered I liked the way helping injured individuals made me feel. This gave me insight into the physician's point of view.

At the same time, I discovered other things about myself. Sports fine-tuned the eye-hand coordination I had found to be a personal strength in wood shop and art class at school and in building model after model at home. My cousin, Dick Geis, who had been a mentor to me and had attended the same college as I did, entered medical school. More than a cousin to me, I believed Dick set an example worth following. I too began to consider medical school.

About this time, two developments were occurring in medical practice that would shape my career. One was the emergence of sports medicine as a recognized subspecialty, and the other was the increasing acceptance and practice of arthroscopy in orthopedics. Arthroscopy is a type of surgery described as "minimally invasive." It is called that because rather than making a long incision on the outside of the knee so that they can see inside, surgeons use an arthroscope. This instrument, with a diameter hardly greater than that of a pen, has within it a camera lens and a fiber-optic light source. Using this "scope," as the instrument is commonly called; the surgeon can see what is within the knee on a television that receives the transmission from the tiny camera lens. By making other small incisions and inserting instruments, the physician can surgically repair what is wrong.

Patients favor minimally invasive surgery because it usually does not require hospitalization, recovery and return to activity is quicker than with "open" surgery, and it is associated with few complications and minimal scarring. Surgeons who excel at performing it have fine motor skills and better than average eye-hand coordination, skills I had begun to hone in school and sports. Today, about three of every four patients I see come to me with knee injuries, some of which are resolved with arthroscopy, some without.

Since my earliest job as co—team physician with the University of Missouri and working with Glenn McElroy, M.D., I have been lucky to have many fine coaches and athletes call me when they needed help. From being team physician at the first football game played in China, to being a physician at the Goodwill Games, to being team physician for Bela Karolyi's Olympic gymnasts, I have found being a sports medicine specialist extremely rewarding. It built on my experience as an athlete, and I found my empathy and understanding of the athlete's predicament could work with his or her desire to return to training or competition to synergize the recovery process. This kind of collaborative effort epitomizes the best of the physician-patient relationships.

But it is easy to understand why professional or Olympic athletes would invest all they had in recovery and rehabilitation. I also wanted this book to expand that type of relationship and commitment. What I had in mind was sharing a conditioning and maintenance plan for ensuring better knee health and preventing injuries in anyone, whether an athlete who punished the knees with constant running on the basketball court, a computer whiz who neglected knee conditioning with sedentary hours at the screen, or anybody in between. Certainly with baby boomers solidly in middle age, a need exists for good prevention advice about avoiding overuse injuries and maintaining strength and flexibility. I've found, too, that many of them, especially as they become caretakers of elderly parents and observe firsthand the price of immobility, are ready to make a commitment to better health. Answering that commitment is also a major objective of this book.

Finally, long ago it became clear to me that there were remedies never taught by Western medical schools that met the needs of patients. I believed their benefits, even if observed in only a few cases, needed to be shared. Perhaps my being part Native American made me more accepting of complementary therapies. When I first started this book more than a decade ago, remedies outside the mainstream were disparaged, especially those provided by non-physicians. Risks were great, critics said, and benefits were unproved. But even in 1991, Americans were spending more than $13 million on such treatment, and in 1993 the conservative *New England Journal of Medicine* published a report on alternative medicine that indicated one in three Americans had tried an unconventional therapy.

Now, of course, many so-called alternative therapies have found haven in major medical centers and medical schools' standing and continuing education curricula. One of the earliest centers for alternative medicine was established in a hospital affiliated with Harvard Medical School. In addition, a National Institutes of Health center established to investigate alternative therapies' worth has celebrated its tenth anniversary, and major insurers include coverage for many of them. However, I'm not suggesting, despite the appeal of their low cost, embracing any and all "natural" labels and closer provider relationships. Risks should be recognized along with benefits, and Western medicine's proven expertise should never be forsaken for risky and unproven "cures." Perhaps *complementary* and *integrative* describe the best use of these therapies; especially as Western medicine applies rigorous testing that substantiates their strengths, making it easier to confirm appropriate uses and to identify wider applications. I want to encourage an openness to new therapies and a respectful consideration of what patients and colleagues, and physicians and non-physicians find useful.

Acknowledgments

Patients have been some of my best teachers. They have taught me what is important to them, what worked and did not work, and each one has helped me be a better doctor to each one that followed. Listening to them, I came to better understand what makes sense and how I could best help them and others. Whether they were professional or Olympic athletes, high school athletics participants, or weekend warriors, they have all inspired and helped shape my practice as a physician. They have sharpened my skill in making appropriate and specific responses in the most complex situations, in fact refining much of my medical school—acquired skill into operating and examining room instinct.

Laying the foundation for that informal but invaluable education was the training I got at the Orthopedic and Fracture Clinic in Eugene, Oregon. There, Doctors Donald D. Slocum, Robert L. Larson, Stanley L. James, and Kenneth M. Singer introduced me to the whole gamut of orthopedic practice and taught me what it meant to be a doctor. Their influence shows up regularly in my practice today, even now, over twenty years after spending one year under their guidance.

Producing any good book requires a collaborative effort between an author and editor, and medical editor Beth W. Allen has reminded me, like a friendly trainer, what the book needed to get in shape and stay in shape. For that, I'm grateful. Professor Kathleen Gibson of The University of Texas Dental School brought her medical anthropology skills to the review of an early version of the chapter on knee evolution and made helpful suggestions. Others along the way made other recommendations that, once incorporated, helped forge the final version you hold.

Foremost, my wife, Allison, is responsible for the completion of this project. She was the number one person urging me to move forward. Her expertise as a dietitian and her experience working in a major medical center made her a valuable contributor as well as a knowledgeable reviewer during the book's evolution.

Black Elk, the Sioux leader, said, "Everything an Indian does is in a circle, and that is because the power of the world always works in circles, and everything tries to be round." With the completion of this book, a line of learning, practicing, teaching, and sharing comes full circle, and all those who contributed—these and many others—stand within its compass.

To my parents, Pauline and Francis Jensen

I

Introduction: The Miracle Knee

*"Human walking is a risky business. Without split-second timing
man would fall flat on his face; in fact with each step he takes,
he teeters on the edge of catastrophe."* —John Napier
"It is better to die on your feet than to live on your knees."
—Attributed to Zapata

*O**ne young Olympic gymnast I treated sustained a stress fracture a few
weeks before the 1996 Olympics in Atlanta. When I explained the
bone-stimulating treatment that had been chosen, I told her she had
an important role to play during the recovery. I described the time she was to
undergo therapy every day as a quiet time, a time to visualize the healing. I
encouraged her to imagine the bone-forming cells (osteoblasts) at work depositing
new tissue and maturing and hardening into osteocytes that would heal the
fracture, creating a restored bone, rich in calcium, magnesium, and phosphorous.
This technique is not unlike the visualization efforts of pediatric patients with
cancer who are encouraged to imagine their immune cells gobbling up cancer
cells like Pac Man swallows his enemies. Not every visualization results in an
Olympic gold medal, but this dedicated young athlete, aided by the unflagging
support of her parents and coach, her youth, and a healthful diet enriched with
additional but not excessive multiple vitamins and minerals, went on in a few
weeks to become one of the members of the gold medal—winning U.S. Women's
Gymnastics Team. Her youth was a bonus not only because she was healthy and
extremely fit but also because she was open to the possibility that focusing on
healing could better the energy producing bone-stimulating treatment and ready
her for world-class competition.*

The most complex joint in the human body, the knee, can elevate
you to king of the world—or at least king of the marathon—or it can,
with kneeling and bowing, place you in homage to those around you. If

you have ever had a knee injury or ever studied anatomy, you probably have marveled at its mechanics.

A Divine but Natural Phenomenon

Crisscrossing ligaments, articulating bones and cartilage, synovial membranes secreting lubricating fluid, tendons of muscles, and friction-erasing bursa all converge at this minimalized ball-and-socket joint—to do what? To create the miracle of movement—to make fluid human locomotion, whether fast or slow, possible. Moving the year-old child from the floor to its mother, sending the shopper through the store stalls, launching the penitent to seek forgiveness, propelling the runner around the Olympic track. Bearing the weight of its owner's body multiplied by the force of that body in movement, the knee is a divine but natural phenomenon that when working well is taken for granted. But when the knee is injured or malfunctioning, its loss can escalate annoyance to grief and evoke a pain and discomfort beyond that attributable solely to the injury.

The knee is second only to the ankle in vulnerability to bone or ligament injuries, and knee injuries cause much greater impairment. More than half of the American population participates in sports activities every year, and of these participants millions will experience a knee injury. In fact, 19.4 million visits to physician offices in 2003 were because of knee problems. Even among those who are not participants in sports, conversations about aches and pains often center around knee injuries of their own, their peers, or their athletic heroes.

The knee is the fulcrum on which is determined superiority or inferiority, resistance or submission, strength or weakness. Because walking upright sets humans apart from their nearest living relatives, the knee's characteristics have been crucial in anthropological studies to identifying which family—human or ape—newly discovered fossils belonged. To be "upright" is to be superior, literally and figuratively.

Conversely, for thousands of years, the bent knee has indicated submission. As a gesture of respect, some children are taught to curtsy, bending their knees and sometimes lowering their heads. People of all ages around the world kneel to demonstrate submission to their god, and many kneel to indicate reverence for religious or political leaders or religious icons. Language symbolically reflects this thinking. Problems of all sorts—emotional, financial, and political "injuries"—"bring us to our knees."

This well-worn and symbolically charged joint, whose surface is familiar geography to every schoolchild, quickly develops in the womb despite its complexity. The eight-week embryonic development of the human proceeds from head to toe, so to speak, meaning that the arms develop before the legs. When the embryo is less than one-fourth inch and only about twenty-four days old, an arm "bud" develops, followed within two days or less by the leg "bud." When the embryo is not yet three-quarters of an inch, the femur, tibia, and fibula appear and the kneecap is evident. When the embryo is about forty-one days old, but still less than an inch long, the knee zone is formed. Within four more days, the knee ligaments appear, and within two more—with the embryo at the ripe old age of forty-seven days—the knee clearly resembles that of an adult.

Though this embryonic development is unbelievably rapid, the knee's history stretches back about 320 million years.

Evolution of the Knee

Three hundred twenty million years ago there lived *Eryops,* an amphibian with a long mouse-like nose, a short bulky body, and a thick but tapering lizard-like tail, which is thought to be the common ancestor of not only today's reptiles but also modern birds and mammals. *Eryops* had knees whose basic characteristics can be found in those knobby protrusions you find in between your thighbones and your shins. Similar to your knee, the knee of the *Eryops* had two rounded projections at the knee end of the thighbone (the femur), which were for articulation with another bone, a relatively flat surface, or plateau, at the top of the shinbone (the tibia). The common characteristics of knees between most extant tetrapods have led some scientists to speculate that *Eryops* even had cruciate ligaments, asymmetrical collateral ligaments, and menisci more than 300 million years ago, just as human knees do today. Those ligaments are the strong bands of tissue unifying your thighbone to your shinbone and are known to many of us through news accounts of athletes who have torn them in play. The menisci are fibrous crescents in between those bones, absorbing the inevitable shocks.

Only four major changes occurred over the next 320 million years to give us the superior joint we call the knee. If you think of these 320 million years being laid out on a football field, with each foot approximately equaling a million years, three of the four changes occurred on one half of the field—in the most recent 170 million years. (You have to keep in mind that there were no modern humans—*Homo sapiens*—in North America until well within the last half inch of the figurative football field, when Cro-Magnon peoples crossed from Siberia and ventured southward into the American plains by way of western Canada.)

The Jurassic Knee

The first change occurred 180 million years ago during the Jurassic Period, when the femur angled in toward the midline and brought the knee's orientation to the front. With this change, walking became more efficient. The next event occurred in the Cretaceous period, during the time of the emergence of the earliest mammals (protomammals). The fibula (the outer and smaller of the two bones between the ankle and the knee) moved farther away from the front and farther below the joint line. The next two changes came at the extremes of the Cenozoic Era, the current geological era. First was the development of the bony kneecap (the patella), about sixty-five to seventy million years ago and not in a common ancestor but apparently in reptiles, mammals, and birds independently. Second was the development late in the Cenozoic Era of the bipedal gait in humans' ancestors. This change incorporated a deviation of the femoral epiphysis from the general angle of the long bone itself, making it possible for the knees to come closer to midline.

To understand this in crude terms, think of how we imitate the gait of an ancient creature in telling a story: "BOOM, BOOM, BOOM," we say to the preschooler, as our heads go side to side abruptly. That's because we think of the legs as coming straight down, much as the legs of a robot or those in a child's primitive drawing do, without any indication of the angulation of the bone from the hip to the knee.

In chimpanzees, walking upright produces the same back and forth movement because the thigh bone does not angle toward the midline as it does in humans. To keep their balance and stay upright, they must move radically side to side to keep their center of gravity over the weight-bearing leg. As with the robot, their wide-apart feet generate what might be called more properly a bipedal *waddle* rather than a *walk*.

Though all four changes over the last 300 million years are extremely important, so are the constants. The striking similarities between the knees of diverse species remain astonishing. The knee has worked for more than 300 million years with few anatomical changes despite dramatic changes in functional demands.

Why Walk Upright?

The question of when hominoids began to walk on two limbs rather than four is being defined by new fossil discoveries by anthropologists, but the question of why humans became bipedal may be more difficult to answer.

The prevailing theory has been that early ancestors of humans—those who lived in trees—were pushed onto the open savannah by climate and environmental changes that forced them out of the trees and onto the ground. Less vegetation meant traveling farther for food and relying more heavily on their wits. A bipedal gait was more efficient and better suited to this life out in the open than was walking on all fours. This theory was supported by environmental evidence indicating that other species common to harsh, open land environments were found in multitudes with the fossils of early bipedal hominids and that evidence of forest-loving animals was largely missing. Then, more evidence, this time from *plants* and *animals,* indicated that these early hominids lived near plants that flourished in a forest and near animals with extremities meant for forest life.

Other theories about the advent of bipedalism have included the theory that being upright made it easier for early humans to see across a plain and theories that humans needed free hands for gathering food, for holding children, and/or for carrying food back to a base camp. These theories feature either men as hunters, women as gatherers, or man as a "provisioner" who was improving his chances for his clan's persistent survival by supplying a mate with food who would in turn produce offspring more frequently. Another theory proposed that shifts in the availability of food forced wider foraging, making bipedalism attractive. A chimpanzee is only about half as efficient walking on all fours (what anthropologists call "knuckle walking") as he would be walking bipedally. So walking on all fours did not have an energy advantage.

Whether the human line became bipedal to free the hands, to hold children or provide provisions for them, or to gather food or avoid becoming food for predators, it is important to remember that humans are the only species that walks with a functional bipedal gait, despite the many similarities between the human knee and those of many animal systems.

That is partly why watching children learn to walk is such an excruciating but deeply cheering experience. Walking is at once one of the most fundamental aspects of being human yet one of the most difficult skills to master in very early childhood. It is as though in gaining the ability to walk, the child obtains much more than the ability to put one foot in front of another.

The Physiology of Walking

The physiology of walking is a complex combination of muscles and bones that requires demanding coordination. The knees' main actions are bending (flexion) and extension, and both are intrinsic to walking.

The hamstring muscles bend, or flex, the leg, and quadriceps muscles straighten, or extend, the leg at the knee. The hamstring muscles are three muscles at the back of the thigh—the semimembranosus, semitendinosus, and the biceps femoris—that make flexing and rotating the leg possible. The quadriceps, made up of four muscles of the front of the thigh, extend the leg for walking. The four quadriceps muscles are the rectus femoris, vastus lateralis, vastus intermedius, and the vastus medialis. These muscles attach to the top of the patella (knee cap) by the quadriceps tendon. The knee cap attaches to the upper front of the shin (tibia) by the patella tendon. The sartorius, gracilis, semimembranosus, and semitendinosus muscles are flexors of the knee. These four muscles also influence internal rotation of the tibia and protect the knee against rotary and valgus stress.

During normal walking the hamstrings are not at rest, but are working, bending the knee. The contraction of the muscles of the lower limbs propels the woman or man or child in walking or running. In between the tibia and fibula of the lower leg is the interosseous membrane that separates the muscles of the front and back of the calf. Plantarflexors at the back of the calf and the quadriceps at the front of the thigh contract in coordination to straighten the leg, bend the foot at the ankle, force the foot's sole (plantar surface) against the ground, and propel the body forward.

A Remarkable History

It takes a multitude of forces to translate muscle activation into locomotion. What forced us to choose bipedal locomotion and what developmental transformations made that possible may only slowly— or never—completely unfold from excavations of our past. What is clear and what remains is the miracle of every step and the remarkable history behind every bend of the knee.

2

Promoting Knee Conditioning and Injury Prevention

"A wise man should consider that health is the greatest of human blessings." — Hippocrates

ary Yanker in his Complete Book of Exercise Walking *tells of a personal experience that taught him the value of stretching before walking. While on a long-distance walk that lasted several weeks, Yanker determined that he wanted to increase his distance from twenty-five to thirty miles per day. To save time, he decided to forsake the four basic stretching exercises that he had practiced faithfully for the previous weeks. The result? By the third stretchless day he had shin splints, the painful tightening in the lower leg when the balance between the muscles of the front and the back of the calf gets out of whack. The pain slowed him to about half his former pace, so the distance he was able to cover was cut in half rather than being increased. "Believe me," he wrote, "it's a helluva way to learn a lesson about the importance of warming up and cooling down for sessions of exercising, whether walking, running, or whatever."*

The security system you buy for your home or car, the safety precautions you teach your children when they are small, the diet changes you make to keep your cholesterol down, all are efforts to preserve what you have and prevent a loss. Certainly some losses can never be recovered, and of those things that can be replaced, the process is rife with hassles, disappointment, grief, and pain. The same may be said of the loss of use or physical ability owed to injury. Ask anyone injured on a playing field who has had to have surgery.

Never simple, never easy, prevention is recognizing and anticipating a potential threat and acting ahead of time to stop or dampen its effect. In terms of your body and your knees, the engine of prevention is conditioning. Conditioning knees so that they can handle the stress put on them is the only way to prevent knee problems or limit their scope. It requires remaining aware not only of the knees but also of the whole body. The body sends out a warning signal (like the flashing light on your dash) that it is being overtaxed when you have run too many miles, hiked too many trails, or practiced too many jump shots. The ability to appreciate this signal comes from performing what might be called a "body check."

Body Check: Getting in Touch with Your Body

A body check, a brief mental and physical evaluation of well-being, involves being in touch with and aware of your body. Foremost, it is a mental awareness of your activity. For example, prolonged knee bending, called *flexion,* and twisting while bearing weight are known to be stressful to your knees. Therefore, if you anticipate having to sit for a long time on a car trip or in a movie theater, for example, realize that this prolonged bending may cause discomfort. Break this constant pressure by extending your leg. Take a walk, sit on the aisle where there is room to stretch out, or find some other way to extend your legs. Knee pain may also come from muscles connected to your knees. Remember, your thigh muscles move your knee, so notice if they are tight. You may need to stretch them throughout the day with quadriceps, hamstring, or calf stretches.

Always perform a body check before you exercise. Here's how it works. Start your stretching routine with, let's say, toe touches. Bend over, keep your knees locked, and reach for your toes. Since everyone's baseline flexibility is different, know what your usual "warmed-up" state is. If you can normally touch your toes and you can touch them now, there is no need to stretch longer or farther. However, if you are only able to get, let's say, one foot from the ground, you need to spend some time stretching to get to a normal stretched-out state. You do this the following way:

Bend over, relax, and slowly reach for your toes. Feel the muscles you are stretching (in this example, the back of your thigh and lower back). Don't bounce. Just gently stretch. The reason not to bounce is that bouncing activates the muscle stretch reflex that causes the muscle to contract. If you can now touch your toes (or reach your normal stretch) and you feel adequately stretched but still tight, stop the stretch.

This means that you need to start the exercise (at one-half speed) and then restretch. When you start to exercise, the muscle gets warmer, and your body responds to this by sweating. Thus, when you start feeling the sweat, it is a good signal that you can stretch a little more vigorously to achieve your maximum stretch. If you are stretched to the max, you can do your exercise or activity full speed. Your warm-up is complete. However, if you're still not stretched out, be careful. You should modify your workout or you could get injured.

Some overall stretches are very familiar to us. When we roll the head gently to the right full circle and then to the left in the same way, we can hear the creaking and popping of the stretching. Afterward, a sense of relaxation replaces the tension formerly there. Another exercise, standing with legs slightly bent and inhaling slowing and deeply while raising the arms over the head and exhaling as you lower them, slows the respiration and helps relieve stress.

Stretches good for your knees and the muscles around them are the calf stretch, the quadriceps stretch, the hamstring stretch, trunk stretches, and groin stretches (see illustrations). Try to hold each stretch at least six seconds, and work toward holding each for 30 seconds.

Calf stretch. Against the wall, place the left toe and elbows and palms of both hands. Place right leg behind left leg with heel down. Press hips into the wall with leg straight. While maintaining stretch, bend knee of right leg, and feel the stretch move down into the heel. Reverse positions and repeat.

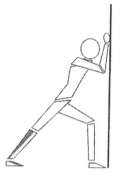
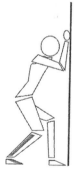

Quad stretch. Kneel on the floor, keeping the back straight. With right hand, hold toes of right foot, pulling ankle toward the body and pushing hip forward. Repeat with other hand and foot.

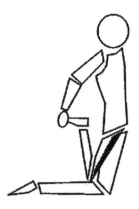

Hamstring stretch. Place heel on a ballet bar or any waist-high object. Bend nose to knee, keeping back straight. To stretch muscles more, bend leg on which you are standing.

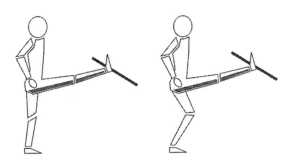

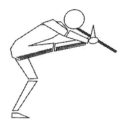

Trunk stretches. Lie on back in tight ball, having pulled bent knees to chest *(A)*. Overhead, extend legs and arms *(B)*. While sitting, raise one leg and twist body while crossing the leg over the other. Repeat with other leg *(C)*.

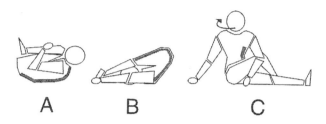

Groin stretches. Sit on floor with legs in diamond shape in front of you. Lean forward to stretch groin and gluteus maximus. Pull heels in close to body, and lean forward, pressing down on knees to stretch groin and inner thigh. Then, with legs straight out to the sides, bend right ear to right leg, and then bend left ear to left leg. Finally, lean forward, pressing chest to floor.

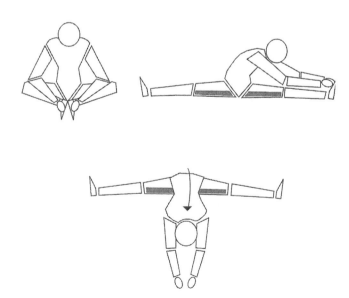

Good activities to aid your knees in warming up are gentle biking (about 60 rpm), walking (3 mph), slow jogging (jogging is "slow" when you can pass the "talk test," which is being able to speak easily while running without becoming breathless), and performing leg lifts.

Flexibility and Strength Training

Warm-up stretches are the foundation of flexibility and strength training and a base on which injury prevention depends. Stiff, inflexible tissues are much more likely to sustain an injury. But some people even overdo stretching—working at it too long or too hard—and injure themselves, all the while having only the best intentions. Stretching should not be a competitive sport.

But stretching is important because even muscle training, like negative factors such as aging or injury, cause muscles to tighten, and this change has to be counterbalanced with stretching. Because the term "strength training" conjures up images of muscle-bound weight lifters, it seems odd to say that it begins with learning to relax. But it does.

Relaxation exercises release tension and allow muscles to stretch. With a combination of relaxation and stretching comes the flexibility that permits a full range of motion at your knees and other joints. Having this full range of motion and the strengthened muscles around the joints not only enhances performance but also provides protection from injury in sports. Furthermore, muscle strengthening improves posture, improving carriage and buffering the threat of back pain. For greater knee strength, try the following exercises: the quad wall sit, hamstring curl, hip flexor or extensor, hip adduction and abduction, and hip extension.

Quad wall sit. This is like sitting in a chair but without the chair. With your feet away from the wall, lean against the wall, back flat. Slide down until knees are flexed and thighs are parallel to the floor. Lower legs should be straight up and down.

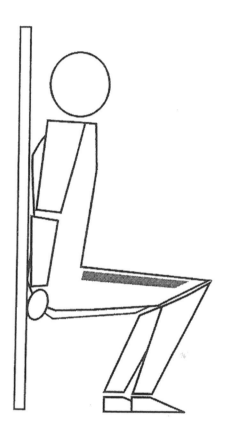

Hamstring curls. Using ankle weights, bend knee and lift leg behind. Repeat on the other side.

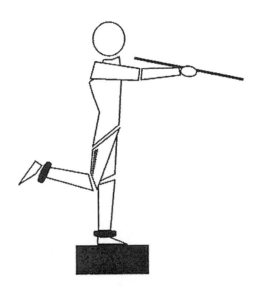

Hip flexor or extensor. With weight on ankle, lift leg behind, keeping the leg straight. Repeat with other leg. To balance muscles, perform the leg lifts forward, lifting toes toward ceiling.

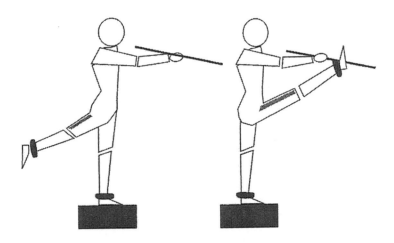

Hip adduction and abduction. This exercise requires a stretchable band attached to the wall. Stand with side to the wall. Put band on ankle nearest wall, move leg nearest wall across other leg, keeping back straight and leg straight *(left)*. Turn around and repeat on other side. To balance opposing muscles, keep band on ankle and move outside leg away from wall *(right)*. Turn around and repeat on the other side.

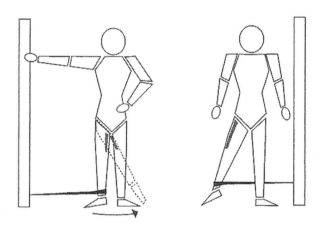

Hip extension. The hip extension exercise should be performed without arching the back. Lie with trunk on table, legs extended to ground at table's edge. Raise legs, holding on to table, until back is straight and legs parallel to floor.

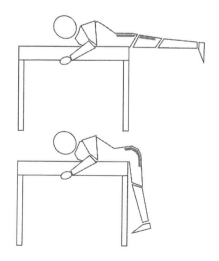

Prevention
Conditioning and prevention are teammates. As conditioning goes up, oftentimes the risk of injury goes down. Having a heightened sense of your body's relative position and improving your ability to move with agility will help prevent injuries.

The ESP of Conditioning: Proprioception
With this increased muscle conditioning comes proprioception. Proprioception is that perception provided by sensory nerve terminals within muscles and tendons that tell the brain about the position and movement of the body. Having a sense of where your joint is helps, and it is why some players never hurt their knees. This is in part because they know where their knee is in space in relation to other objects. They don't leave it exposed, sticking it out of the football pile-up, for example, to get shattered. In skiing, proprioceptive athletes give and fall when they feel the possibility of tension starting in the knee. The old adage that knowing how to fall is as important as knowing how to stay up is correct. If you are a beginning skier, remember to spend some time practicing how to fall safely on the ski slope.

Preventing Knee Injuries by Improving Agility
Agility drills are another way to prevent knee injuries. Not only do they strengthen the muscle fibers to fire more quickly, they also hone the proprioceptive sense. An easy drill is to start a slow jog and then progress to a faster pace. When you are comfortable with your pace, start making some large figure 8 turns. When these come easily, decrease incrementally the size of the figure 8. Finish by making sharp cuts to the right and left. This drill may take a few minutes or a few weeks; progress may be slow if you have been injured.

Stairs and Steps
Running the stadium steps has been a standard for some school athletes for conditioning, and some coaches prescribe it as a disciplinary penalty. We now know this is punishing to your knees and specifically your kneecaps if not to your spirit. The problems it causes are threefold. The first is that eccentric contraction of the muscle (downhill running) causes muscle soreness. The second is that knee flexion with weight puts extra pressure on the knee and kneecap. The third is that this is an "open-chain" activity. A "closed-chain" activity keeps your foot on something (biking is a simple example and machine stair climbing, leg

pressing, or skiing are others). When you jump or take your foot off a platform and reposition it, an increased force is applied, which may be many times your body weight. Therefore, a combination of all three of these can cause trouble with stairs.

One step program has devised something called an "air bench," which has a flexible wood platform over a spring meant to absorb impact and protect joints. It even puts spring in your step with the resulting reaction from the impact.

However, just as a sip of wine doesn't cause alcoholism, a moderate amount of traditional stair stepping, bench work, or other similar activity is OK. The only patients I tell to avoid open-chain activities are ones who have pain while doing them (that's a no-brainer) and those with knee problems.

Bench aerobics probably got their start because of boredom with a pure dance aerobic workout coupled with a desire to get a more demanding workout. As I stated above, too much can bring men or women to their knees, but a moderate amount of bench aerobics is OK. Maybe many men and women doing aerobics had not experienced the negative aspect of running stairs in football and basketball, and a step program appealed to them. It was known to be a quick way to raise the heart rate and get a better workout. The Harvard step test is a standard way to medically "stress" someone (a patient is rapidly stressed by a step regimen, and heart rate and blood pressure are recorded and compared to average, or normal, values). As step programs gained popularity, athletes and doctors contributed advice from their experience and better workouts resulted. Using a lower step goes a long way toward preventing injury and decreasing the power of the three drawbacks mentioned above without diminishing the aerobic effects of the workout.

Running

What about running and your knees—is it bad? An offshoot study of the famous Harvard Paffenberger study of cardiac disease and lifestyle was a study on knees. This study showed that running did not necessarily cause knee problems unless you already had a problem. A moderate amount of running doesn't cause problems if you don't have an existing mechanical problem. We are genetically designed to be able to run to catch food, to evade our enemies, and to survive. In fact, our genes and bodies aren't that radically different from those of early humans; however, because of various reasons (technology, for one), we have become out of shape and overweight and bring biomedically incorrect stress to our knees.

Runners may be categorized into four groups. The first group is comprised of those who are disabled and can't or shouldn't run as a mode of exercise. Running may put force on the knee that may cause or increase arthritis. The second group is made up of those who are temporarily disabled. Being overweight may be the problem. Exercise should be of minimal impact to start (swimming, biking, or using weights, for example), and it should progress to running very slowly. If you increase your exercise more than ten percent per week, you may develop knee pain. A sure-fire way to kill the desire to continue an exercise program is overmotivation and undertaking a program too vigorously too soon.

The third group of runners run a moderate amount—three to five times per week for twenty to forty minutes each time, or around three miles at each outing. I just do not see these people in my office with injuries. Fortunately, the American College of Sports Medicine recommends working out three to five times per week at two-thirds your maximum heart rate for thirty minutes. This is a sufficient workout and won't hurt you.

Six-time Ironman Triathlon Champion and Personal Trainer Mark Allen recommends calculating your maximum heart rate using these guidelines:

1. Start with 180 and subtract your age
2. Subtract another 10 if you never exercise, or
3. Subtract another 5 if you are an occasional athlete, working out less than 3 days per week, or
4. Leave the number alone for an athlete who has trained consistently 3-4 days per week for the last several years
5. Add 5 beats if you are over 60 or under 20 years.

The number you end up with will be your maximum aerobic heart rate. If you exercise below this rate, you will burn fats for energy. If you exercise above this number, you will burn carbohydrates. Both systems are important, but the fat burning one is the one that takes the longest and is the most difficult to develop.

The fourth group of runners is comprised of those who exercise compulsively. These are patients who have to exercise. They generally keep exercising even in the face of knee pain. I'll never forget the patient who always had knee pain at mile twelve. I asked him why he didn't just run eleven miles, and he said he never thought of that option! Again: moderate exercise can make your knee pain go away. You may have a minor mechanical abnormality that doesn't become a limiting factor and initiate pain until a certain stress level is exceeded.

The American Running and Fitness Association endorses a twelve-week plan of walking and running that provides an easy start and plenty of cardiovascular workouts over the long haul (see table).

Easy 12-Week Walk/Run Program!

	DAY ONE	DAY TWO	DAY THREE	DAY FOUR	DAY FIVE	DAY SIX	DAY SEVEN
1	Walk 15 min. Vary your pace. Try not to stop.	Walk 5 min. Run 1. (Repeat for a total of 17 min.) Walk 5.	Walk 15 min. Vary your pace. Try not to stop.	Walk 5 min. Run 1. (Repeat for a total of 17 min.) Walk 5.	Walk 15 min. Vary your pace. Try not to stop.	Walk 5 min. Run 1. (Repeat for a total of 17 min.) Walk 5.	Rest!
2	Walk 15 min. Run 1. Walk 2.	Walk 5 min. Run 3. (Repeat for a total of 21 min.) Walk 5.	Walk 15 min. Run 1. Walk 2.	Walk 5 min. Run 3. (Repeat for a total of 21 min.) Walk 5.	Walk 15 min. Run 1. Walk 2.	Walk 5 min. Run 3. (Repeat for a total of 21 min.) Walk 5.	Rest!
3	Walk 15 min. Run 1. Walk 2.	Walk 6 min. Run 4. (Repeat for a total of 26 min.) Walk 5.	Walk 15 min. Run 1. Walk 2.	Walk 6 min. Run 4. (Repeat for a total of 26 min.) Walk 5.	Walk 15 min. Run 1. Walk 2.	Walk 6 min. Run 4. (Repeat for a total of 26 min.) Walk 5.	Rest!
4	Walk 15 min. Run 2. Walk 4.	Walk 3 min. Run 2. (Repeat for a total of 30 min.) Walk 5.	Walk 15 min. Run 2. Walk 4.	Walk 3 min. Run 2. (Repeat for a total of 30 min.) Walk 5.	Walk 15 min. Run 2. Walk 4.	Walk 3 min. Run 2. (Repeat for a total of 30 min.) Walk 5.	Rest!
5	Walk 15 min. Run 2. Walk 4.	Walk 5 min. Run 5. (Repeat for a total of 35 min.) Walk 5.	Walk 15 min. Run 2. Walk 4.	Walk 5 min. Run 5. (Repeat for a total of 35 min.) Walk 5.	Walk 15 min. Run 2. Walk 4.	Walk 5 min. Run 5. (Repeat for a total of 35 min.) Walk 5.	Rest!
6	Walk 30 min.	Walk 4 min. Run 6. (Repeat twice.) Walk 5.	Walk 30 min.	Walk 4 min. Run 6. (Repeat twice.) Walk 5.	Walk 30 min.	Walk 4 min. Run 6. (Repeat twice.) Walk 5.	Rest!
7	Walk 30 min.	Walk 4 min. Run 6. (Repeat twice.) Walk 5.	Walk 5 min. Run 10. Walk 5.	Walk 4 min. Run 6. (Repeat twice.) Walk 5.	Walk 5 min. Run 10. Walk 5.	Walk 4 min. Run 6. (Repeat twice.) Walk 5.	Rest!
8	Walk 30 min.	Walk 2 min. Run 1. (Repeat 9 times.) Walk 5.	Walk 5 min. Run 15. Walk 5.	Walk 2 min. Run 1. (Repeat 9 times.) Walk 5.	Walk 5 min. Run 15. Walk 5.	Walk 2 min. Run 1. (Repeat 9 times.) Walk 5.	Rest!
9	Walk 30 min.	Walk 1 min. Run 30 sec. (Repeat 20 times.) Walk 5.	Walk 5 min. Run 20. Walk 5.	Walk 1 min. Run 30 sec. (Repeat 20 times.) Walk 5.	Walk 5 min. Run 20. Walk 5.	Walk 1 min. Run 30 sec. (Repeat 20 times.) Walk 5.	Rest!
10	Walk 5 min. Run 20. Walk 5.	Walk 15 min.	Walk 5 min. Run 20. Walk 5.	Walk 15 min.	Walk 5 min. Run 20. Walk 5.	Walk 15 min.	Rest!
11	Walk 5 min. Run 25. Walk 5.	Walk 15 min.	Walk 5 min. Run 25. Walk 5.	Walk 15 min.	Walk 5 min. Run 25. Walk 5.	Walk 15 min.	Rest!
12	Walk 5 min. Run 30. Walk 5.	Walk 15 min.	Walk 5 min. Run 30. Walk 5.	Walk 15 min.	Walk 5 min. Run 30. Walk 5.	Walk 15 min.	Rest!

GET ACTIVE!

It's easy. Here's how...

√ Check with your doctor when starting to run. This is especially important if you or your family have any heart problems, high blood pressure, high cholesterol, breathing problems, diabetes, or if you are overweight or smoke.

√ Get well-fitting, well-cushioned running or cross-training shoes. If you run less than 10 miles a week and don't have a history of sports injuries, most entry-level running shoes will work for you. A specialty shoe store with knowledgeable salespeople can help you find a shoe made for your needs. Or send a self-addressed, stamped envelope to American Running to get our Running Shoe Database Questionnaire.

√ Wear comfortable, loose-fitting clothes. If the temperature is cool, dress in layers so you can strip down as you warm up.

√ Ask a friend to join you. When getting started, it sometimes helps to find a friend to work out with. You'll motivate each other.

√ Schedule time for your workouts — mark it on your calendar. If you set aside a definite time to exercise, you'll be more likely to keep the commitment.

√ Keep a log. You'll be surprised and proud of how much you are doing. It also makes it easier to track your progress.

In the twelfth week of the program, you will be running about three miles without stopping, depending on your pace. Following the association's suggestions for making the program work will increase the chances that you will achieve the results you want:

- Get your doctor's OK.
- Get well-fitting, well-cushioned athletic or multipurpose

shoes. (When you're running twenty minutes a shot invest in moderately priced running shoes.)

- Wear comfortable, loose-fitting clothes. Dress in layers to strip down as you warm up.
- Make a firm appointment with yourself for each session, and keep it. Don't make excuses; if you think you'd rather nap, don't! Get moving instead. You'll be glad you did.
- Find a friend who will join you on your workouts. In getting started, it sometimes helps to have a friend run with you. You'll motivate each other.
- Keep a log. You'll be surprised and proud of how much you are doing.
- Brag a little. Other exercisers at all levels will applaud you, and couch potatoes will respect you. They may even emulate you.
- Listen to your body. If you are sore, skip a session.
- Take stock. At the end of week two, see if you aren't feeling better, more energetic.
- Take a look. See if there isn't a healthier, more vigorous, better looking you in the mirror.

Walking

Walking is a great exercise for your knees. Walking is a total body exercise because you use your arms, back, and legs. Therefore, you need to get in shape to start a walking program, and the best way to do it is to stretch and start walking!

Among the benefits walking enthusiast and author Gary Yanker cites for walking are its low cost (no expensive or special equipment, clothes, or memberships required), its practically injury-free practice, its naturalness, its easy modification to a wide variety of styles and speeds, its circulatory benefits, and its usefulness as a bridge to other sports. Added to this must be the mental health benefits of being outside, breathing fresh air, and physically leaving behind the reminders of daily life stresses.

Although it is true that no special equipment need be purchased for walking, the importance of choosing an athletic shoe that properly fits your foot and serves your purpose should be emphasized (illustration).

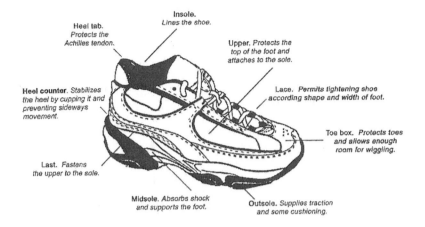

Insole. *Lines the shoe.*

Heel tab. *Protects the Achilles tendon.*

Upper. *Protects the top of the foot and attaches to the sole.*

Heel counter. *Stabilizes the heel by cupping it and preventing sideways movement.*

Lace. *Permits tightening shoe according shape and width of foot.*

Toe box. *Protects toes and allows enough room for wiggling.*

Last. *Fastens the upper to the sole.*

Midsole. *Absorbs shock and supports the foot.*

Outsole. *Supplies traction and some cushioning.*

Choosing an Athletic Shoe

Understanding the parts of an athletic shoe can help you choose the right shoe and prevent problems you may have experienced with other shoes. The aim is not to recommend a specific shoe manufacturer but to help you be a knowledgeable consumer. After all, athletic shoe prices can put a dent in the monthly family budget (the most popular shoes cost from $45 to $135), and ill-fitting shoes can transform a pleasurable activity into a painful one. A good rule of thumb is to match your scrutiny and cash outlay to the intensity of your running shoe use. If you are having trouble with your shoe fitting your foot, you may find that using two laces, choosing a shoe with a specific kind of eyelet, or adding a removable liner may help.

The Sole

The sole is made up of the *outsole,* the *midsole,* and the *insole.* The *outsole* is the bottom of the shoe. Made of different components, the outsole is most commonly made of black Eva. Manufacturers try to match sole treads to specific sports. To prevent slipping and to gain traction, choose the tread with the most waffling and rippling. As its name implies, the *midsole* lies between the outsole and the insole. Air or Eva or other material is used here for cushioning. The less the materials will compress, the better they are. The *insole,* or inner lining of the shoe, sometimes now comes with more padding on the medial, or inner, side of the shoe. After some wear, inserting a new liner provides renewed shock absorption. Spenco and Viscolax are brands whose liners are less heavy than Sorbothane.

The Upper

The *upper* is the material on top of the shoe. Mesh or nylon breathe and are lighter than leather. Don't make the mistake of thinking your shoe won't need replacing until the upper shows wear. Shoes usually lose their shock absorption long before the upper wears out.

The Last

Binding the upper to the sole is the *last*. The upper may be fastened to the sole in one piece (slip-lasted) or may be fastened to a full-length fiber board (board-lasted). Others may be fastened to a fiber board in the heel and sewn in one piece around the front of the foot (combination-lasted). Depending on your arch, your pronation, the straightness of your foot, and the speed at which you will be running, you should get a shoe with a straight last or a curved last.

Other Characteristics

Choosing a shoe that is wide enough in the *toe box* (the space in the shoe for the toes) means the toes should have sufficient height and width for comfort, including a finger's width of distance between the toe and the end of the shoe. The lack of adequate space in the toe box of many women's dress shoes explains why women have bunions more frequently than men. Above the toe box, in the metatarsal area, the foot also needs adequate space, but a shoe that fits here and in the toe may be too loose at the heel. To solve this problem (one often encountered by women), buy an athletic shoe that is manufactured in various widths, choosing the one that best fits. Lining the heel with moleskin tape can reduce movement on the heel, as can using the extra high eyelets some manufacturers put on some shoes. Plastic eyelets will help you tighten the shoe around the foot. Using two shoestrings, one on the lower eyelets and another on the upper ones will also help compensate for differences in fit between the front of the shoe and the back. A padded *heel tab* protects the back of the Achilles tendon. Notching in the heel tab gives the tendon room to move when the toe is down but the sole is perpendicular to the floor. The *heel counter* stabilizes the heel by preventing side-to-side movement and helps decrease overpronation (painful flat-footedness). Some shoes have a doubled heel counter to maximize heel stability.

There are many walking shoes on the market and some running shoes will work. You want a stable rear heel counter and a firm but cushioned sole. You can give yourself and your knees a quick new shoe by replacing the insoles. Replaceable insoles such as those made by Spenco can take significant force off your knees.

Getting the Most Out of Your Walk

Some people use hand-held weights called Heavy Hands and/or ankle weights to walk. Research shows that squeezing the weights in your hands increases your workout and thereby your heart rate. Nonetheless, I have reservations about both. I don't recommend ankle weights because they put too much abnormal force on the knees. High school kids use them, but kids of that age seem to tolerate about anything. If you are going to use arm weights, I suggest weighted wristbands. They are easy to use, and you don't have to hold on to them. Of course, vigorous pumping of your arms can also help. A word of caution about race walking—it is a sport in itself. Be aware of the significant increase in torso twist and other movement that is different from simply walking fast.

Fast walking can be better for your health and knees rather than slow jogging. The reason is that the average person walks most efficiently at three and one-half miles per hour. When you need to go faster, you automatically break into a slow jog (imagine speeding up on the sidewalk to catch the green light). This transition comes so naturally because your body "knows" it is more energy efficient to jog slowly than to walk fast. Therefore, use knowledge of this physiological accommodation to your advantage. You *want* a workout, so it's OK to be energy *in*efficient and thereby increase your heart rate. The fast walk doesn't put nearly as much force on your knees as the jog—another benefit.

Cross Training

Cross training is imperative for good knee health. Cross training is athletic conditioning or drills employing different activities, mixing, for example, a central activity with one that rests, or unloads, the body from stresses of the main activity. When we were hunters-gatherers, our physical activities were very diverse. As modern-day foragers more likely to graze in a mall than in a field, we don't get enough exercise in our normal routines, so we need to exercise perhaps not to accomplish necessary work but maybe still to survive! However, any specific exercise if done repetitively can cause an overuse injury. Pain on the inside of a knee can be just overuse—"runner's knee" or "breastroker's knee." The treatment I prescribe for overuse is what I call "cross training" or "active rest." You need to stay active but need to rest the area that takes the most stress in the primary activity. Activities fall into weight-bearing and non-weight-bearing categories. If your main activity is walking or running, you need a cross training activity that is non—weight bearing such as swimming or biking. Some activities are closed-chain and minimally weight bearing (Nordic Track, stair stepper, leg press).

Beating the Weekend Warrior Syndrome

When you undertake a conditioning program for greater flexibility, strength, and range of motion, you will discover yourself having a better mental outlook, improved endurance, and fewer injuries, especially those brought on by overuse or imbalanced muscle groups. Knees, which often bear the brunt of a self-generated "weekend warrior" triathlon of increased high-impact exercise, gardening, and home repair, can be partly protected from these injurious enthusiasms by the conditioning options outlined in this chapter. Whatever options you choose, make sure your approach to conditioning is one you enjoy and can perhaps share with others. Walk or run with an office buddy. Join a class with a friend. This will better ensure that you will enjoy it and will make it an integral part of your life.

3

Fueling Your Body's Performance

"You are what you eat."—Adelle Davis

A forty-five year-old professional came to me with complaints of knee pain. He had a meniscus tear that required arthroscopic surgery. The only barrier to performing the repair was the fifty extra pounds he was carrying that was likely to cause arthritis in the injured knee.

He had never considered the burden his extra weight was to his knee. The knee on a person of average weight can support three times the body's weight during normal, brisk walking or stair climbing. Playing sports, jumping, running, or pushing the knee's limits in any way raises the demand. Every extra pound puts an extra burden on the knee, every step of every day. In his case, he was adding an extra 150 pounds of pressure with every brisk step.

Intervention: consultation with a nutritionist. A three-day reckoning of his every bite produced convincing evidence of how he had gained the weight and revealed a pattern he could change to reverse his gain to loss. Making sure that he understood basic facts about foods and the impact of choices, that he was ready to change his behavior, and that he was willing to undertake a modified exercise program I devised to avoid further injury to his knee, convinced me he would taste success. Losing weight not only made him look and feel better and decreased the chance of postoperative arthritis, it also improved his sense of well-being and decreased his risk for heart disease, high blood pressure, and diabetes.

Relax. This is not a lecture on the food pyramid. What it is, is some information about nutrition that's pertinent for any person who is on the go and realizes the health of any part, including the knee, depends on the health of the whole.

In the first part of this chapter, the role of diet, the various nutrients (and how much of each is needed), vitamin supplements, and fluid replacement during exercise are topics. Then the focus will shift to diet and weight control. There's a big difference between controlling weight and controlling body fat. What needs to be emphasized is how to listen to the body and how to approach diet change slowly and successfully.

The Role of Diet in Health

The best advice about making the most out of food is to forget fads. There is no magic diet that will transform an average person or even an above average person into a star. Diets don't create strong, agile bodies; strength and agility come only through training. But diet gives the body the raw material it needs to construct the body that is desired. So diet must be complete.

Look at it this way: an automobile assembly line would have a hard time turning out cars if it had no wheels or windshields, never mind how flashy the leather interior or how radical the instrumentation. A good diet has to include all the essential nutrients or the "car" won't run.

The U.S. Department of Agriculture's experts on diet and nutrition summarize their recommendations for healthy eating into seven dietary guidelines, which are meant for every American age two or older:

- Eat a variety of foods. Eating a broad array of foods is important to ensure that bodies get all the calories, protein, vitamins, minerals, and fiber they need to stay healthy.
- Eat in moderation so that obesity is avoided. Maintaining a healthy weight helps avoid high blood pressure, diabetes, heart disease and stroke, and certain cancers.
- Choose a diet low in fat to help maintain a healthy weight. Keep fat, saturated fat, and cholesterol to a minimum to help reduce the risk of heart disease and certain cancers.
- Make vegetables, fruits, and grain products, all of which are generally lower in fat, mainstays of your everyday diet. They provide vitamins, minerals, fiber, and complex carbohydrates.
- Minimize sugar intake. Sugars add calories, few nutrients, and promote tooth decay.
- Minimize salt intake.
- Drink alcohol in moderation.

How Much of What?

The body needs six kinds of nutrients: carbohydrates, proteins, fats, vitamins, minerals, and water. Carbohydrates, proteins, and fats give you energy, while vitamins, minerals, and water keep the body machinery humming to deliver that energy. They support the enzymes and hormones that carry out the chemical reactions that make everything happen.

Carbohydrates, proteins, and fats are the "crude oil" from which the body's gasolines—glucose and fatty acids—are refined. Glucose is a special form of sugar that comes from carbohydrates and proteins. Fatty acids come from proteins and fat.

In simple terms, about 60 percent of daily calories should come from carbohydrates, 15—20 percent from proteins, and the rest (20—25 percent) from fat. Below are suggested practical ways of achieving this balance.

Exercise and Fuel

The two forms of exercise—aerobic and anaerobic—use the body's fuels in vastly different ways.

Aerobic exercise

Aerobic is an adjective used to describe something that needs oxygen to exist. When used to describe a kind of exercise, it indicates that the exercise conditions the heart and lungs, making oxygen intake ever more efficient. The muscles use oxygen slowly enough to allow the blood to continually replenish the supply. Breathing is hard, but hasn't advanced to gasping. (If a person can't talk during the exercise, it's not aerobic.) Aerobic exercise burns fat and some sugar.

Pure sugar does two things: *(a)* it gives an immediate but short energy boost, and *(b)* it increases the insulin level. Insulin is the enzyme that the body uses to burn sugar for energy. The extra insulin created by aerobic exercise burns up all the sugar and then looks around for more, making you feel hungrier than ever. Even worse, the increased insulin blocks the enzymes that make fat available as fuel, so the fat campfire starts to go out! Depressing, isn't it?

Anaerobic exercise

Anaerobic is an adjective used to describe something existing in the absence of free air or oxygen. In anaerobic exercise, the muscles have essentially used up all the free oxygen and the blood cannot deliver enough in time. Without oxygen, the muscles can't burn fat; they are forced to find some other fuel. The alternative the muscles select is glycogen, a stored form of sugar. Some glycogen is warehoused in the muscles themselves, making it an easily accessed energy supplement.

Other glycogen resides in the liver; however, for it to get to the muscles, blood must carry it there. In anaerobic exercise, the muscle is already working so hard that the blood supply is not adequate; therefore, liver glycogen is not a viable long-term solution for anaerobic energy needs. In desperation, the body burns muscle to meet its energy needs, which is not a great solution if the aim is to build more.

The President's Council on Physical Fitness and Sports has identified running; bicycling; basketball, handball, or squash (they are rated equally); and skating or cross-country skiing as the best sports for assisting in weight control. In the table are listed activities and the estimated calories they demand per minute.

Table 3.1. Physical Activities and Caloric Demand

Activity	Calories/Minute
Cross-country skiing	10–15
Jogging/running	10–12
Canoeing or rowing	3–11
Handball, squash, or racquetball	6–11
Swimming (crawl stroke)	8–10
Jumping rope	7–10
Biking, tennis, ice or roller skating	3–10
Aerobic Dancing	4–8
Walking	5–7
Golf (walking with clubs)	5
Ballroom dancing	4

Components of a Complete Diet

Carbohydrates

Carbohydrates are the breads, cereals, rice, and pastas that form the foundation of the food pyramid, and experts recommend six to eleven servings daily. Typical serving sizes include one slice of bread, one ounce of breakfast cereal, or one-half cup of pasta. Carbohydrates contain the sugars and starches necessary to keep the body running and the fiber necessary to ensure smooth functioning. One gram of carbohydrate yields four calories.

The body converts sugars and starches to glucose for energy or glycogen for energy storage. Fiber keeps the intestines running well and helps prevent constipation, heart disease, cancer of the colon, and diabetes. (Do not look down on the lowly bran muffin.) About 60 — 65 percent of the calories in your diet should be carbohydrates. Contrary to popular opinion, potatoes alone will not make you fat. Only the butter, sour cream, and cheese that make them taste so good do that.

One question that always arises regarding carbohydrates is whether an athlete should "load carbos"—eat large amounts of carbohydrates— before a competition when demand on the muscles will be greatest. The idea behind carbohydrate loading is to force the body to store extra glycogen in the muscles so that the glycogen can supply energy in endurance events. People have developed elaborate schemes to turn carbohydrates into muscular glycogen. Most of these schemes include exercising to exhaustion (or fasting) to deplete glycogen stores and then tanking up on spaghetti and other carbohydrates. But fasting or exhaustion exercise can be very hard on the body. It may cause more damage than any possible benefit obtained from loading up afterwards.

The food eaten immediately before an event does not generally improve performance—superior performance comes from the dietary and training habits of the past several months. The meals right before a strenuous competition should not contain high-protein or high-fat foods. They take longer to digest, they increase the stress on the kidneys, and they may fail to supply the needed nutrients because of demands made on the blood supply by stress and tension on the day of competition. The best meal is one rich in carbohydrates, whether the exercise is to be intense or prolonged. Athletes should allow three hours for proper digestion and absorption of this carbohydrate-loaded meal.

Here are some guidelines:

- Eat solid food three to four hours before the event, or drink a liquid meal two to three hours before. The liquid meal should be low in fat and protein and have some vitamins and minerals.
- Avoid anything that causes gas. You don't need jet propulsion.
- Don't eat sweets or sugared drinks within one hour of the event. The insulin they stimulate will eat up the glycogen.
- Be sure to drink enough to stay hydrated.

Proteins

Foods that build tissue and muscle and repair cells, proteins are the only food compounds that contain nitrogen. When these proteins break down during digestion, they provide the amino acids needed to manufacture a seemingly infinite number of special-purpose proteins, including enzymes, hormones, and even structural components of body cells. A protein's measurement in energy is the same as that for carbohydrates (four calories). The ever-resourceful body can use proteins for energy by converting them to fatty acids or glucose.

Proteins come to us in meat, fish, eggs, beans, nuts, and dairy products. Vegetables have proteins too, but are called "incomplete" proteins because they do not contain every amino acid. That is how vegetarian diets can lack important nutrients.

Only 10 –15 percent of all calories an average person eats daily should come from protein, which amounts to two or three servings a day. A serving equals two to three ounces of meat, poultry, or fish; an egg; or one-half cup of cooked beans. Because the body cannot store it as protein, it is converted into a stored energy source: fat.

Although athletes may need a little more protein than non-athletes, the protein consumed in the typical American diet exceeds the protein needed. Supplying the body with more than it needs is hard on the kidneys besides being hard on the waistline. Balance is important: if a diet is not balanced and even if calorie intake is too low, the body will use protein for energy rather than for building muscle. This is why carbohydrates are so important.

Sources of vitamins and minerals as well as proteins and carbohydrates, vegetables bring variety to any diet for good health. Along with them, fruit contributes vitamins, minerals, and sugar. Oranges, grapefruit, tomatoes, and strawberries are rich sources of vitamin C, and pumpkin, carrots, apricots, and cantaloupes are good sources of vitamin

A. Broccoli is a good source for both. Though vegetables can provide many proteins the body needs, they are considered an incomplete source of protein because they cannot provide all of the amino acids, the building blocks of protein. Of the necessary amino acids, the body can manufacture all but nine, and these, called the *essential amino acids,* must come from diet. Vegetarians combine incomplete proteins, pairing beans with corn tortillas or beans with rice, for example, to achieve a complete protein. Or they combine an incomplete protein, such as pasta, with a complete one, say a milk product such as cheese.

Fats

Fats include many categories. One you've heard about is cholesterol, one of the sterols. The major storage form of fats is triglycerides, which consists of glycerol and three fatty acids. One gram of fat yields nine calories. This is the body's favorite way of storing energy because it is so efficient. To lose one pound of fat, more than twice as many calories as are in one pound of glycogen or protein must be burned.

Fats appear mostly in foods we love: ice cream and chocolate, plus meats, eggs, whole milk, cheese, fried foods, butter, margarine, salad dressings, oils, and mayonnaise, to name a few. Brussels sprouts have no fat.

Diets with high fat intake are associated with being overweight or obese and having heart disease and diabetes. Fat intake should not exceed 20 – 25 percent of total calories. A gram of fat supplies more than twice the calories of a gram of carbohydrate or protein. Not fair, is it?

Vitamins

The Food and Nutrition Board of the National Research Council states that a proper mix of foods should provide adequate amounts of vitamins and minerals. Nonetheless, it is probably a wise safety measure to take a multiple vitamin supplement every day.

Now, some people think that if a little is good, a lot will be better, so they take megavitamin doses. These regimens are probably not helpful; in some cases it simply creates very expensive urine, in others it is dangerous.

Water-soluble Vitamins

The key water-soluble vitamins are B complex and C vitamins.

Too much niacin from a B-complex vitamin can cause fatigue, tingling, skin flushing, and liver damage. Megadoses of the other water-soluble vitamins do not appear to be toxic because the body simply rids itself of the overload by dumping the excess vitamins into the urine.

Fat-soluble Vitamins

Fat-soluble vitamins are a different story. These are vitamins A, D, E, and K, and they remain in your body, especially in your liver, until your body uses them. If more than is needed is consumed, they accumulate and toxic symptoms result. In fact, too much vitamin A can be deadly.

Minerals

Minerals fall into two categories: major and trace. The human body requires relatively large amounts (more than 100 mg a day) of major minerals, including calcium, iron, magnesium, potassium, and sodium. Of the trace minerals, including chlorine, chromium, copper, fluorine, iodine, manganese, molybdenum, phosphorus, selenium, sulfur, and zinc, little is needed. Generally speaking and excepting calcium, iron, zinc, and potassium, supplements of the minerals aren't necessary.

Calcium strengthens the bones of which your knees are made and all other bones and teeth as well. It also aids in the clotting of blood, the signaling of nerves, and the contracting of the heart and other muscles. It also protects against osteoporosis. Some studies have found that calcium (1,200 — 1,500mg/day) helped reduce the risk of colon cancer in patients who had had colon polyps removed. Such polyps are generally recognized as early precursors of cancer.

The general recommendation is for 800 mg for men and women 25 years of age or older, but a National Institutes of Health Consensus Panel used 800 mg as a baseline and recommended higher doses, especially for older adults and women who are pregnant or breast feeding.

Table 3.2. *Daily Calcium Requirements by Age Group*

Group	Calcium Needed (mg/day)
Children 1–10 years	800–1,200
Young adults 11–24 years	1,200–1,500
Adult women to age 50 years	1,000
Women 50 years and older	1,500
Women who are pregnant or lactating	1,200–1,500
Adult men 25–64 years	1,000
Men 65 years and older	1,500

If you eat enough dairy products (i.e., drink at least three to four glasses of milk a day), you should get enough calcium. There are 300 mg of calcium in a cup of low-fat milk. If you hate milk, consider low-fat yogurt (415 mg/cup), Mozzarella cheese (550 mg/ounce), or calcium-fortified orange juice (300 mg/cup). Otherwise, take a calcium supplement. Some nutritionists recommend taking calcium supplements at night because of better absorption.

Many young Americans are not getting the calcium they need. In a 1999 survey reported by the Centers for Disease Control, only 18 percent of high school—age students reported drinking three or more glasses of milk per day during the seven days preceding the survey. Furthermore, milk consumption fell as age increased in both girls and boys, with lower classmen being significantly more likely to have drunk three or more glasses than were upper classmen.

Menstruating women should eat plenty of iron-containing foods (for example, spinach, flank steak, figs, turkey, baked beans, pork loin) or take an iron supplement, since iron is the absolutely critical part of the hemoglobin in the blood. Hemoglobin carries oxygen; without enough oxygen circulating, you won't have the energy you need.

Zinc, important in maintaining a healthy immune system, is required in moderate amounts daily. The recommended dietary allowance (RDA) is 15 mg/day for men and 12 mg/day for women 19 years of age and older. Women who are pregnant or breast-feeding require between 15 mg/day and 19 mg/day. According to the National Institutes of Health, six ounces of beef chuck offers 90 percent of the RDA.

Potassium is a salt-like sodium that your body loses when you sweat. Foods rich in potassium include bananas, orange juice, and cereals. Taking a small daily supplement of potassium might be wise.

Water

The human body is 65 percent water, and it just doesn't work well with less. Fluid lost during exercise must be replaced. In normal activities, most people do not suffer a water deficiency.

In heavy exercise, though, an athlete "burns" sugar and fat for energy. When fuel is burned, heat is generated, just like a wood fire produces warmth. If a body doesn't get rid of that heat, it can cook to death. That's what happens when people have heat stroke. Sweating keeps you from getting too hot. The water cools the skin as it evaporates from it. But with every drop, the ability to cool is diminished. Dehydration reduces the body's ability to dissipate heat and impairs endurance.

Weighing yourself before and after exercising helps indicate how much water the body has yielded to keep cool. Drink two cups for every pound lost.

How sweat Works

The main way the body gets rid of heat is to sweat. Why does this work? Because it takes a lot of heat to turn water from a liquid to a vapor. (Just think of how long you heat a pot of water before it boils.) Your body cools itself through the vaporization of sweat. Every drop of sweat that evaporates carries heat with it.

Normally, a person in an hour-long aerobic dance class will burn about three hundred calories, and the heat will be carried off by about a pint (two cups) of sweat. People who exercise harder (like competitive athletes) burn more calories and generate more sweat.

Water Replacement

To sweat, the body must have water within it. So those who exercise must continually replace water lost during a workout. As little as two percent dehydration will impair the body's ability to regulate temperature, and at only three percent dehydration, muscles lose endurance ability, according to McArdle, Ketch, and Ketch in *Exercise Physiology* (Lea & Febiger, 1986).

Complicating water replacement is the movement of blood to the muscles, leaving the digestive system little power. If a lot of water is consumed during exercise, the body may have a difficult time taking advantage of the available pool. A better idea is to load up before a workout, and then to take a few sips every few minutes as needed. It is unlikely that this will mean more trips to the bathroom—this water will be used for sweat, not urine. In addition, making sure the water is cool will further help ensure against overheating.

Special "Exercise" Fluids

But what about sports drinks that replace "lost electrolytes"? Medical reports leave experts divided on the use of these supplemental drinks. They may be useful when someone who is exercising has overextended himself, and his sweat begins to taste salty. A longer or heavier or faster workout may make demands on the body that these drinks can meet, since they provide both sodium and potassium. Supplements with sugar should not be necessary unless the workout extends more than one hour at a stretch.

For athletes engaged in endurance events, experts have recommended adding carbohydrates to fluids to bolster fluid replacement with the carbohydrates, which are meant to sustain the concentration of blood glucose and help ensure carbohydrate oxidation throughout the event. Practical recommendations include monitoring weight loss as an index to water depletion (each pound lost corresponds to about 15 ounces of lost water and replacing it with fluids at about 80 percent the rate of sweating). For endurance events, experts have estimated that both carbohydrate and fluid needs can be met by ingesting 19 – 38 ounces of fluid per hour containing four percent to eight percent carbohydrate.

Diet and Weight Control

Two variables control weight: diet and exercise. To lose weight, a person must employ both. Too much emphasis on one or the other, and balance is distorted. Anorexia and bulimia are two conditions of extreme dieting that result when balance is lost.

Watch Out for That Diet

Anorexia nervosa is a condition that is both psychological and physical. Patients with this condition find themselves unable to eat, even when their bodies are starving. They think about food or dieting constantly and obsessively, they feel fat despite objective proof of the opposite, and they want to lose weight even when there is no indication they should. Left untreated, anorexia can result in death.

Patients with bulimia, like those with anorexia, are obsessed by food, but rather than refusing it, they eat uncontrollably and then force themselves to vomit or take laxatives to avoid gaining weight.

Both of these patterns are extremely damaging to the body and deprive the body of necessary vitamins and minerals.

Fat Control and Weight Control

Weight is easy to measure, but it is not a very good way to determine body fitness. Weight includes bone, muscle, water, fat, and other tissues. But obviously those who have most of their weight in muscle are much better off than those who have most of their weight in fat, even if they weigh the same.

Because muscle weighs more than fat, a person can be building muscle and trimming down the size of his or her body and be gaining weight at the same time. Obsessing about weight can lead to depression when the same changes should lead to elation.

The best way of keeping tabs on your body is to monitor your percentage of body fat. Unfortunately, there is no such thing as a body fat monitor you can step on every morning in the bathroom. Body fat can be measured three ways: immersion in water, skin fold measurement by calipers, and electrical impedance. The immersion method is the most accurate, but quite complex and expensive. Calipers measure the thickness of skin folds in certain areas of the arms and abdomen. The thickness depends on the amount of fat under the skin, which is a good indication of total body fat. The electrical impedance method measures the flow of a tiny current of electricity through the body and uses a computer to calculate body fat. The "standard" amount of body fat for a "normal" adult female is 26 percent; for a male, 15 percent. Athletes have less.

A Nutrition Plan That Works

A nutrition plan will only work if you personalize it to your needs and your likes and dislikes. Some recommended diet may be wonderful, but if broccoli is a big feature and you cannot stand broccoli, forget it.

The best plan is to analyze the current diet and take a close look at what goals are to be attained. Then making small, gradual changes makes it easier to migrate to a healthy eating style that can be maintained for a lifetime. The main thing is to avoid another dreadful diet. Instead, the goal should be to figure out how to eat healthfully.

It is a myth that the less one eats, the faster one will lose weight. Starving only makes a dieter hungrier, and sooner or later he or she will compensate by going on a binge. Then the dieter will feel guilty and starve himself or herself even more...and so on in cycles.

Evaluating the Present Diet

Looking honestly at current food choices will require keeping a food diary. For four days, a would-be dieter should keep track of what and how much he or she eats—including what is eaten weekend days as well as weekdays. For each meal, what was eaten and how much should be recorded, and snacks should not be forgotten. Then summarize the results:

- Ounces of meat per day. Three ounces is equivalent to one regular hamburger, one chicken breast, one chicken leg (thigh and drumstick), one pork chop, or three slices of pre-sliced lunchmeat.
- Servings of breads and cereals per day, preferably whole-grain. One serving is one slice of bread, one ounce of cereal, or one-half cup cooked cereal, pasta, rice, or grits.
- Fruit. One serving is a whole piece of fruit, one-half cup juice, one-half grapefruit, one-quarter melon, one-half cup cooked or canned fruit, one-quarter cup dried fruit.
- Vegetables. One serving is one-half cup cooked or chopped raw vegetable or one cup leafy raw vegetable.
- Cheese per day or week. One serving is one ounce. Note whether it is low fat or regular.
- Milk per day. One serving is one cup. Note whether it is skim, low fat, or whole.
- Egg yolks per week.
- Lunchmeat, hot dogs, corned beef, sausage, bacon, other highly processed meats per week.
- Baked goods and ice cream (cake, cookies, coffeecake, donuts, etc.).
- Servings of snack foods per day or week (chips, fries, party crackers).
- Spreads used per day. One serving is one pat of butter or one tablespoon of salad dressing.

Guidelines for Healthy Eating

After the food diary has been kept for four days, the results should be compared to the guidelines below for a healthy diet. These are daily requirements.

- Two to three servings of meat, for a daily total of about six ounces. This also includes eggs, though you should limit your eggs to four per week. Dried peas and beans can be substituted for meat.
- Six to eleven servings of bread, cereals, rice, or pasta, preferably whole-grain products.
- Two to four servings of fruit.
- Three to five servings of vegetables.
- Three to four servings of dairy products, which should be low fat.
- Three or fewer margarine or other "spread" servings.
- Minimal snacks and sweets.

A healthy diet will have little obvious fat in it. No mounds of chips and crackers or pounds of cheese. (Most people don't realize that cheese is about 75 percent fat). You won't see gallons of ice cream either, or baskets of French fries, or bags of fast food. Even when people set out to avoid fat, most diets will still have enough to meet nutritional needs.

Eating wisely may sound very difficult to achieve, but the trick is to take it one step at a time. No one achieves perfection overnight—that isn't possible. Instead, the aim is to establish healthy eating habits that will stand the test of a lifetime.

Developing a Success Strategy

Once a baseline is outlined (the analysis of current eating habits) and a goal is set, anyone can build a sensible eating plan. Remember that no plan is cast in concrete. Chances are modifications will be necessary as the plan is implemented, based on what works individually.

At least 60 percent of calories should come from carbohydrates (that's complex carbohydrates like vegetables, cereal, and pasta—not sugar); 10—15 percent from protein; and no more than 25 percent from fat.

Eliminating all the fun foods can make a diet unbearable. Sometimes having a small piece is better than saying no altogether to that piece of Chocolate Decadence Double Fudge Cake. Think about the amount of food eaten, not just what the choices are.

Below are some tips to make getting started easier.

Listen to Your Body

The single most important thing about eating sensibly is staying in touch with the body while eating. Some people get so obsessed with counting calories, they lose the ability to tell when they are hungry or full. Overweight people typically continue to eat when they are not hungry, especially at night.

To cope with the urge just to put something down the hatch, dieters should ask themselves the following questions:

- Are you really hungry? Or are you bored or angry or lonely? Eating cannot help any of these other problems.
- Are you eating in a hurry? Eat slowly to give your body a chance to absorb the food—that's the only way it can tell you when it's had enough! Stop eating when you feel comfortable, not when you feel full.
- Have you reminded yourself that food is close by somewhere? If starvation feels imminent, you can always eat again.
- What makes you hungry? How much of what makes you feel comfortable? How long does a certain type of food "stick with you"? Use your diet as a tool. Practice it. Experiment.
- What is motivating you to eat so much? Forget that stuff about "cleaning your plate." Mothers have been saying that for centuries (along with the part about starving children). That's a terrible way to learn how to nourish your body.
- What do you crave? When you crave an orange, go eat one! Our bodies are very clever in telling us what they need, if we're clever enough to listen.

Day-in, Day-out Choices

If you are determined to change your wayward ways in favor of weight watching, you must also identify your daily fat allowance. Experts recommend that the general population get no more than 30 percent of daily calories from fat. Currently, the average person in the United States gets 37—40 percent of his or her calories from fat.

Most processed food has a label showing the number of grams of fat in the food. But each individual must figure out the total grams of fat that are right for him or her.

To calculate daily fat allowance, one must identify how many calories are burned each day. The figure is 2,000 calories a day for a moderately active woman and 2,500 to 3,000 calories a day for a moderately active man. The calories burned depends on age, sex, and quotient of exercise.

The follow equations will help:

$a \times n = fn,$

where a is the percentage at which you want to keep fat intake, n is the number of calories, and fn is the number of calories from fat. Then

$fn / 9 = fa,$

where fn, again, is the number of calories from fat, and fa, is the fat allowance. The number of calories from fat are divided by 9 because one gram of fat provides nine calories. Therefore, a person consuming 2,000 calories per day who wanted to keep the fat allowance to 20 percent of the diet would be allowed 44.4 gm of fat per day:

$.2 \times 2,000 = 400$
$400 / 9 = 44.4$

Once this is calculated, the dieter can carefully read labels and keep fat consumption under 45 gm per day. A fat counter helps teach us where hidden fats lurk. These can often be found at the grocery checkout counter.

Listing the fat content of most foods would take a book in itself, but here are some samples. As can be seen, fat is almost everywhere:

- One tablespoon of salad dressing (or one big pat of butter) contains 13.3 gm of fat (120 calories).
- A large egg has 5 to 6 gm of fat per yolk.
- Two tablespoons of cream cheese (about one ounce) has 10 gm of fat and only 2 gm of protein.
- A quarter—pounder with cheese has about 31 gm of fat. A small quarter-pound hamburger has about 11 gm.
- One raised donut has about 10 gm.
- One-half cup of gourmet ice cream has 20 gm.
- Two slices of bologna have about 15 gm.
- One medium croissant has about 10 gm.
- Three chocolate chip cookies have about 10 gm.

- One ounce of potato chips has about 10 gm.

Some fairly simple measures can make a significant difference in the fat that gets into you. Here are ten from the article "Eat Right, America" published in the *Journal of the American Dietetic Association:*

- Drink skim milk.
- Eat whole-grain breads. Choose one tasty enough to eat without butter.
- Use jam, jelly, or all-fruit spread instead of butter on toast and rolls.
- Eat more pasta, rice, and vegetables.
- Eat lean meat, fish, and poultry. Remove skin from chicken.
- Substitute a vegetable for a meat as an entrée.
- Use low-fat or fat-free salad dressings. The new ones taste fine.
- Snack on carrot sticks, unbuttered popcorn, and unsalted pretzels instead of fried chips, crackers, and cookies.
- For dessert, choose fruit, angel food cake, or sponge cake. Use fruit purées as icing.
- Substitute low-fat or frozen yogurt for ice cream. Try frozen juice bars.

Start with small changes. Identify a fatty food that is easy to eliminate, and do without it. Next week, pick out another. And so on. Don't try to do it all at once.

Keep track of progress. Record the changes made and compare your current status to your goal. Reward any successes. Remember that this is a program of progress, not perfection. This is not a plan to follow until a particular goal is reached but a pattern of living to be made a habit for a lifetime. So keep it pleasant.

Getting Professional Advice

A registered dietitian is an expert who can separate facts from fads when it comes to food and nutrition. Dietitians are at work in many areas of our lives—with food companies, in sports medicine centers, hospitals, health clubs, research laboratories, day-care facilities, and senior citizens' centers.

To locate a registered dietition in your area, log on to *www.eatright. org* or ask your doctor to call the local hospital. You can also write to the National Center for Nutrition and Dietetics, 216 West Jackson Boulevard, Suite 800, Chicago, Illinois 60606-6995.

Finding Balance

Eating a balanced, nutritious diet without too much fat has proven to be a challenge for most Americans. To put what they know about carbohydrates, proteins, fats, vitamins, and minerals to good use—making up a healthful diet—those who want to change must understand that progress and not perfection is the purpose. Further, the overall aim is to change for the better for a lifetime, not just ride the roller coaster of food fads and trends. Listening to signals from the body and approaching diet rationally, one step at a time, bring successes that deserve recognition, no matter how small. Each one affirms the conviction that whether the focus is the part—the knee—or the whole—nutrition—they are inextricably intertwined and neither can be disregarded in understanding.

4

Troubleshooting Common Knee Problems

"Everyone who is born holds dual citizenship,
in the kingdom of the well and in the kingdom of the sick."
— Susan Sontag

*F*irst impressions are generally right. In medicine, evaluations of this sort are sometimes called intuitive diagnoses. When I am examining a patient at my office and I put my hand on the patient's knee, I can usually sense the emotional state of the patient, and that gives me information I need to understand this patient's unique case. In this exchange, I am reminded of the significance of touch not only in healing but also in transferring something spiritual. A priest or minister may place a hand on a baby being baptized, on a child being confirmed, on a couple getting married, or on a candidate entering the ministry or priesthood. This touch communicates grace and a spiritual energy. In medicine, the transfer can be either way: from the physician to the patient or from the patient to the physician. In an initial examination, particularly, the communication is from the patient to me.

Sometimes in such an examination, when I touch a patient's knee, I can sense fear. When I do, I sometimes write that impression down in the margin of the chart or I "file" it in the back of my mind. As I continue through the examination, I may find that everything checks out fine and that anatomically the patient is fit. Then I look again at the complaint: perhaps it is vague. Then I look again at the patient: perhaps in his or her eyes I can see confusion. Then I reevaluate the context. Perhaps the patient is accompanied by a spouse who contradicts the patient's reports. Perhaps the patient is a teen-age boy, accompanied by his mother and father. Perhaps he has a vague complaint about his knee immediately before football workouts are to start. The mother may look worried; the father, impatient. From this, I get a snapshot of the scene and I integrate that scene with the initial impression and the anatomical evaluation. Maybe this boy doesn't want to play football. Maybe he is afraid he is just not *big enough. After performing my evaluation, I make an effort to have patients talk through what they are experiencing. The patient explains how the ailment is limiting movement and where the pain is occurring; I explain different problems, giving the patient an opportunity to identify which ones most closely parallel the complaint that brought the patient into the office. Together we work toward a definition of the problem and solutions to it.*

These situations remind me of Dr. Alfred Schweitzer's positive view of witch doctors, who plied their trade near his African clinic. "Don't expect me to be too critical of them," the missionary physician told visiting Norman Cousins, the author of Anatomy of an Illness as Perceived by the Patient. *Dr. Schweitzer explained: "The witch doctor succeeds for the same reason all the rest of us succeed.... We are at our best when we give the doctor who resides within each patient a chance to go to work."*

When we think of our knees, we tend to think only of the knee surface that we skinned when we were children. We vaguely know the other terms that relate to the knee—*cartilage, ligament, tendon*—perhaps best from the sports pages, but until our knees begin to hurt, we may not bother to understand their meaning. But knowing what makes the knee works helps us understand what is wrong when we have a knee problem, why we are in such pain when we are hurt, and what solutions exist to treat and prevent such discomfort.

A Hinge But Not a Hinge

Like a hinge, the knee permits movement. But one fundamental element is missing. Unlike a hinge, the knee has no pin to connect the leg bones. It depends on an intricate system of interior and exterior bands, special surfaces, and natural shock absorbers to facilitate and smooth the action, to say nothing of keeping the lower leg attached to its upper counterpart. That the knee is more than mechanical parts is best demonstrated by the fact that medical device manufacturers have not been able to devise an artificial replacement that truly reproduces the knee's capabilities.

Four *ligaments* hold the four bones of the leg and knee together. These are dense bands of tissue. *Cartilage* appears in the knee in two forms: covering the surfaces of the bones where they would come in contact with each other and as separate additional buffers. Connecting muscles to the knee and holding the kneecap in place are fibrous cords of tissue we know as *tendons*. Below, beginning with a description of bones and ligaments and moving through their relationship with cartilage and tendons, we will explore the basic mechanics of the knee. Then we'll see how that smoothly running machinery can, like a failing car, lock, grind, grate, and crunch its way to disability. We'll examine why it happens and what you can do about it.

Use the following troubleshooting chart to identify what's bothering you and your knee. Did you have immediate (acute) pain after the injury? Or is a dull pain always present (chronic)? Did your knee swell within the first twenty-four hours or only later? When the injury occurred, did you hear a pop, or do you hear one when you notice the pain? Do your knees lock? Can you sense a grinding, or do they simply give way? Think about where the pain you feel occurs, and use that as a general guide. Then use the chart to narrow down the types of ailments typically related to that kind of pain.

After the chart, you'll find explanations covering common knee and hamstring problems by the location of the pain—the knee in general, the kneecap in particular, the sides of the knee, and the front and back of the knee.

If you need a physician to diagnose your knee ailment, consult "The *Snap, Crackle,* and *Pop* of Knee Injuries" for a list of questions to consider together.

Troubleshooting Common Knee Problems

Diagnosis	Sudden pain	Chronic pain	Sudden swelling (<24 hr)	Late swelling (>24 hr)	Pop!	Locking	Grinding	Giving way
Pain in the Knee in General								
Bursitis	√	√						
Water on the knee		√		√				
Fractures	√				√			
Tumors		√						
Bone and cartilage separation						√		√
Pain in the Kneecap								
Softening of kneecap cartilage		√		√			√	
Kneecap dislocation	√		√		√			√
Pain on the Sides of the Knee								
Runner's knee		√						
Ligament injury	√		√		√	√		√
Meniscus tear	√	√		√	√	√	√	√
Synovial tissue overgrowth and irritation		√		√				
Loose bone or cartilage within the knee		√		√		√	√	
Localized spontaneous osteonecrosis		√						
Pain in the Front or Back of the Knee								
Tendonitis		√						
Hamstring Strain	√		√					
Growth plate inflammation		√		√				
Osgood-Schlatter's		√		√				
Patellar-femoral syndrome		√					√	

The Kneebone is Connected to the Thighbone

The children's rhyme gets us started in the right direction. The knee *is* connected to the thighbone, but it may not be quite as simple as you think. Flexing or extending your knee moves three other bones besides the kneecap; the *femur*, or leg above the knee, connects to the *tibia* (shin) and the *fibula* (nonweight-bearing bone) of the leg below the knee. Protecting this joint is the kneecap, what you can think of as nature's substitute for the pin in the hinge. When you extend, or straighten, your leg, you can feel the kneecap (*patella*) move down the front of the joint. It rides in the *femoral groove,* a depression, or trough, in the lower end of the thighbone. Below the kneecap is the top of the shin, which has a bump on front called the *tibial tuberosity* where the tendon holding the kneecap in place connects.

Keeping these bones connected are not other bones but four ligaments, two within the knee joint (*cruciate ligaments*) and two outside (*collateral ligaments*). The cruciate ligaments cross at the center of the knee and connect the thighbone and the shin. *Cruciate* means "cruciform" or "cross." The stronger of these two ligaments, the *posterior cruciate ligament,* connects from the posterior (back) to the front, and the *anterior cruciate ligament* connects from the front to the back. These ligaments work to prevent the shin's moving forward or backward under the thighbone, hyperextending the knee, or hyperflexing the knee. The two collateral ligaments—the *medial collateral ligament* along the inside of the joint where the knees touch and the *lateral collateral ligament* on the outside of the leg—give the knee stability and work to prevent displacement sideward.

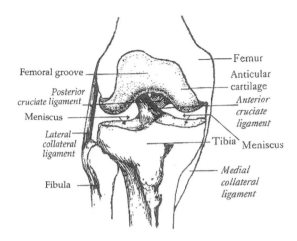

Femoral groove

Posterior
cruciate ligament

Meniscus

Lateral
collateral
ligament

Fibula

Femur

Articular
cartilage

Anterior
cruciate
ligament

Tibia Meniscus

Medial
collateral
ligament

The major bones and ligaments of the knee.

Glide or Grind

Cartilage is what makes the movement of the bones a glide rather than a grind. In the knee, *articular cartilage* is a high-tech protective coating (like Teflon) for the surfaces of the bones facing the joint—the ends of the thighbone and shinbone and the back of the kneecap. Opalescent and somewhat transparent, this smooth, flexible, and in part elastic covering permits easy movement of the joint. Synovial fluid lubricates the system.

But absorbing most of the shock between the thighbone and the shinbone is another type of cartilage. Separate from the bones and different in structure from the articular cartilage, the *meniscal cartilage* buffers the shocks, bears the weight, and protects the bones. Like a washer in a plumbing assembly that has been halved into opposing crescents, two menisci (me-NEH-sky) in each knee surround the joint. They relieve friction and their outer third bears about 70 percent of the weight and shock the knee sustains. The menisci prevent the thighbone and shinbone from wearing on each other and thereby help protect the articular cartilage. The significance of this bit of anatomical engineering is evident in the price paid when a meniscus may be abused and lost because of a knee injury: early onset of disabling arthritis.

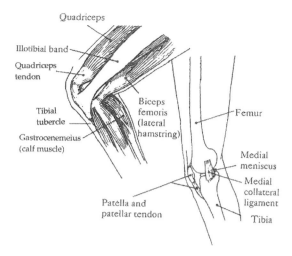

Quadriceps

Illotibial band

Quadriceps
tendon

Tibial
tubercle

Gastrocenemeius
(calf muscle)

Biceps
femoris
(lateral
hamstring)

Femur

Patella and
patellar tendon

Medial
meniscus

Medial
collateral
ligament

Tibia

The tendons of the knee and the kneecap.

Tendons are transmitters. Made of white connective tissue, *tendons* are cords or bands that unite a muscle with a bone and transmit its force, causing movement. The most well-known tendon is the Achilles tendon, which connects the bone in the heel with the muscles in the calf. In the knee, tendons attach to the muscles of the thighs (quadriceps) and the kneecap. The kneecap resists the force of the tendon holding it in place. If the pressure between them remains balanced and no alignment problem exists, the kneecap moves predictably within the femoral groove. If the pressure becomes imbalanced by a sudden event, say, a slip that ends not in a fall but in a jolting recovery of balance, or a long-term training inequity that creates dramatically different strength levels in muscles attached to the tendons, the kneecap can crack or become dislocated.

Locating the Pain

Below are described common knee and related problems by the area where the pain is felt: the knee in general, the kneecap in particular, the sides of the knee, and the front and back of the knee. Some of these are more common to children, adolescents, or young adults (avulsion fractures, bone and cartilage separation, growth plate inflammation, patellar-femoral syndrome) or older adults (localized arthritic condition) than to others.

The *Snap, Crackle*, and *Pop* of Knee Pain

Asking yourself the following questions, writing down your answers, and taking the record to the physician will jump-start diagnostic efforts.

What about pain?

Where do you feel the pain?

When did it start?

Does it recede? If so, when does it return?

Does it worsen with certain movements?

What relieves it? Medication? Rest?

How do you characterize the pain? Numbness? Tingling?

What degree of pain do you feel? Dull ache? Severe, sharp pain? Stiffness?

Does the pain or stiffness limit how you move your knee?

Does your knee *snap, crackle,* or *pop?*

Did you hear an audible *pop* when your knee first failed or hurt?

When you move your leg, do you hear a grating or crunching?

Do you hear clicking when you move your leg? Do you feel it? Where?

Do you feel a grinding in your knee with movement?

Does your knee lock? Catch? Give way unexpectedly?

How does your knee look?

Is the kneecap noticeably misplaced?

Is the knee red? Is it warm?

Is it swollen? When did the swelling begin? Has the swelling increased or decreased? Did both knees swell simultaneously?

Do red lines run up or down from your knee?

How does this problem relate to the rest of your life?

Have you recently increased the amount of time spent exercising or extended your commitment to gardening or home repairs or upkeep?

Have you changed your diet?

Have you been sick?

Did you recently buy new shoes? Have you been wearing very old shoes?

What's your family history?

Has anyone in your family had rheumatoid arthritis?

Are hip joint or back problems present in your family?

Common Knee and Hamstring Problems

General Pain in the Knee

Below are knee ailments characterized by pain throughout the knee system. Bursitis, the first condition reviewed here and commonly called "housemaid's knee," affects many people whose daily work keeps them on their knees—housekeepers, carpet layers, and electricians, for example. In contrast to the gradual toll taken on knees by these careers, unexpected injury in athletics or the impact against a dashboard in a car accident can also cause bursitis. Another familiar condition, commonly called "water on the knee," also causes generalized pain, but it is accompanied by swelling and may require surgical intervention. Other conditions characterized by overall pain are fractures and tumors.

Bursitis

Problem

A bursa, or empty sac, can, after repeated pressure or use of the knee, fill with fluid and become irritated or inflamed (the *-itis* in *bursitis*). Playing football, laying carpet, installing plumbing, or keeping house— any activity or occupation that requires repeated kneeling—can cause the bursa in front of the kneecap to become irritated. When it does, the condition is called *bursitis* or *housemaid's knee*.

Symptoms

Bursitis causes localized swelling, redness, tenderness, and pain. A physician may be able to feel fluid in the sac.

Solutions

If the bursa is extremely irritated, the knee must be immobilized. If it gets redder or hotter and red streaks ascend from the knee, the bursa is infected and antibiotics are needed. In less severe cases, a support or wrap around the knee may ameliorate the condition. Patients can use heating pads and anti-inflammatory drugs to relieve the pressure from the built-up fluid. Addressing the cause of the ailment by reducing the time spent on the knees, using a low rolling stool, or using knee pads (either soft or hard) available at the hardware store will help eliminate or reduce bursitis.

Another solution to an uninfected painful joint is a supplement produced from the antlers of deer. It is relatively new to the U.S. supplement market. Deer velvet, a traditional medicine long used in Asia, is marketed today primarily by producers in New Zealand, where researchers have found trends in data indicating the agent's ability to improve strength and endurance. Available in a powder and a freeze-dried extract, deer velvet has been used to relieve pain and accelerate healing. The annual winter shedding of antlers by deer produces a natural opportunity for harvesting the velvet, causing no harm to the deer.

Water on the Knee
Problem

The synovial membrane lines the knee joint and secretes synovia into the joint cavity. This membrane, like other tissues of the body, can become irritated and inflamed, resulting in chronic inflammation or a chronic infection, depending on the cause. Torn cartilage, joint mice (see section on loose bone or cartilage below), chondromalacia, overuse, and other causes account for these changes. When the membrane is irritated, it secretes more synovia, oftentimes causing the joint to swell, a condition commonly called "water on the knee," or synovitis.

Symptoms

Generalized swelling and pain, from mild to severe, accompany this reaction. Pain can be particularly severe on motion, and no weight may be borne by the knee.

Solutions

Keeping off the knee should help, unless the cause is something other than overuse. If the cause is joint mice (see section on loose bone or cartilage below), the condition may require surgery.

Fractures
Problem

There are essentially three main types of fractures. The first is traumatic fracture from a definite injury. Patients always ask if the bone is cracked, broken, or fractured. If I say the bone is fractured, many times a patient will say, "Oh, thank goodness. I'm glad it wasn't broken." In reality, there is no reason for relief. These terms all mean the same thing. If the fracture is in line and in place, a physician generally will not have to set it or move it into the correct alignment. If it is out of line, the physician will have to correct it to the prescribed alignment. Occasionally, this cannot be done by conservative means (by hands alone), and the patient has to be taken to surgery for anesthesia and a *closed reduction* (*closed* meaning no incision) or an *open* procedure (meaning an incision is necessary) so that the bones may be directly realigned. The bones about the knee are often pinned, screwed, or plated.

A second type of fracture is a stress fracture, which is caused by overloading. The most common stress fracture about the knee occurs in the proximal, or upper, shinbone. This condition may be termed a "march" or "fatigue" fracture. The term comes from the long marches required of new military recruits. Unused to long-distance marches, their leg (tibia) or foot (second metatarsal) bones are soon overloaded. A small microscopic fracture starts and is propagated with every footstep. Eventually this fracture can become quite painful.

The treatment for stress fractures consists of activity changes, allowing time to pass, bracing, and sometimes requiring the use of crutches. Some stress fractures do not heal well, and electrical stimulation may be necessary. It is unusual to have to do surgery or bone grafting to a stress fracture. Tibial stress fractures may require four months to heal, and only then can an athlete run and pound hard on the leg.

An avulsion fracture, the third type of fracture, typically occurs in children. The muscles pull on the tendons, and the tendons are attached to the bone. Many times this bony attachment is not solid because of a growth plate, the flat structure from which a bone grows. Since bones grow from these plates, they are not solid, and these attachment areas are somewhat weak. If there is an abrupt pull, such as one caused from simple jumping, sometimes the force may avulse, or pull off, a piece of bone. If the bone remains relatively close to its original position (for instance, let's say within less than a half inch), we may treat it with a cast or brace. If it has pulled off farther, we may have to reduce it by repositioning the bone without an incision while the patient is anesthetized, or by pinning or screwing the area back. Such was the case with an Olympic gymnast who jumped very hard and pulled off her tibial tubercle growth plate.

Tumors

In a treatment program, a physician must also be sure that pain is coming from the knee. In children and adults, pain in the knee can be associated with low back problems such as herniated disks, hip problems such as arthritis, or a slipped growth plate (capital femoral epiphysis) in the child. Slipped capital femoral epiphysis is a condition in which the growth plate actually slips in the hip area, but generally there is no pain there. Instead, it limits hip motion and brings knee pain. Although no one likes to talk about them, tumors do occur about the knee. In fact, the knee is one of the most common locations in the body for all types of tumors.

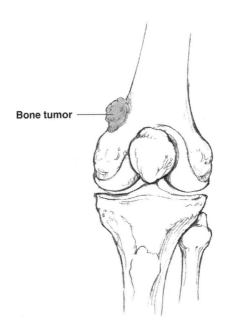

Bone tumor

Bone tumors, such as the one sprouting here from the femur, are rare.

Tumors are either benign—an overgrowth of normal tissue—or neoplastic—what is considered cancer. This second type of growth is definitely abnormal, can metastasize or spread to other areas of the body, and has the potential to be fatal. Many times bumps around the knee are benign tumors called osteochondromas (*osteo* means "bone" and *chondroma* means "cartilage"). Only the larger variety of these has a large cartilage cap with the potential to become neoplastic. There is also a little more worry if patients have multiple osteochondromas throughout their whole body. There are many types of cancers (neoplastic tumors), varying by age group and the tumor's malignancy period. Osteosarcoma is a very aggressive, potentially fatal tumor found in the knee. Any type of knee bump or nodule that does not go away and any radiographically detected abnormal area on the knee should be fully evaluated by a professional.

Bone and Cartilage Separation
Problem

Bone and cartilage separation, or osteochondritis dessicans, is a condition in which the bone *(osteo-)* and cartilage *(chondro-)* aberrantly separate or break off *(desiccare* is Latin for "to dry up"). Its cause is unknown, but theories include a localized impairment of blood supply, unfavorable metabolic conditions, or repetitive trauma. Some experts postulate that it is inheritable. It usually appears without warning in children 6 to 14 years of age.

Symptoms

An achy knee with minimal swelling may be the first symptom, and complaints of the knee's giving way, catching, or locking will follow if the cartilage and bone partially separates. If they totally separate, the patient may rightly sense that a part of the knee is loose inside its framework. Occasionally osteochondritis dessicans is detected on X-ray films taken for other complaints before the child reports symptoms.

Solutions

Exercise, protection, support, and anti-inflammatory drugs are the mainstays of treatment, and sometimes surgery is necessary. When symptoms first appear, such non-weight-bearing exercise as swimming or biking is best to unload the joint, and anti-inflammatory medication should decrease the pain and swelling. Some patients find help in a knee brace or support. A physician may order X-ray films to better identify the lesion and determine if the cartilage and bone have separated. Magnetic resonance imaging also provides this information and can help the physician follow healing after intervention. A computerized tomography scan of the bone can tell how much activity is localized in the lesion. If non-surgical therapy fails to improve the condition, arthroscopic drilling may stimulate the bone to fill in the defect. Sometimes during arthroscopic surgery, the loose cartilage and bone can be reattached with screws or pins. Occasionally, when pieces are loose, they are beyond being reattached and must be removed. After surgery, most patients are able to return to sports and work without difficulty; however, a small percentage goes on to have localized arthritis or wearing in this location.

Pain in the Kneecap

Pain in the kneecap is not only clearly focused, but the condition is also visually identifiable by the misplacement of the kneecap. Sometimes, however, pain in the kneecap radiates, making the pain more general.

Softening of Kneecap Cartilage
Problem

Chondromalacia is the softening of the cartilage, a condition occurring most frequently in the kneecap. The term comes from the Greek word *malakta* meaning "softness." Improper tracking of the kneecap through the femoral groove causes this softening, or degeneration, which is a form of arthritis. Reasons for this improper tracking include a "Q angle" of greater than 20 degrees, uneven strain on the kneecap, poor metabolism in the cartilage causing it to wear away prematurely, or femoral anteversion (a condition in which the knees seem to face each other because the entire leg is turned in at the hip).

The "Q angle" is the angle formed between two intersecting lines: an imaginary line extended from the hip joint, along the quadriceps, and through the knee joint (this is the angled line in the bottom of the capital Q) and a line drawn from the knee cap directly down to the tibial tubercle (the vertical axis). Ideally, the angle is 15 degrees, and any angle greater than 20 degrees indicates increased risk of improper tracking and therefore chondromalacia. Because girls' hips widen as they grow older, their risk of chondromalacia increases as the Q angle widens.

Uneven weight training results in chondromalacia when muscles that have been worked unevenly put uneven strain on the kneecap. In some people, knee cartilage seems to wear out sooner than it does in others, and chondromalacia may be an indicator of this condition.

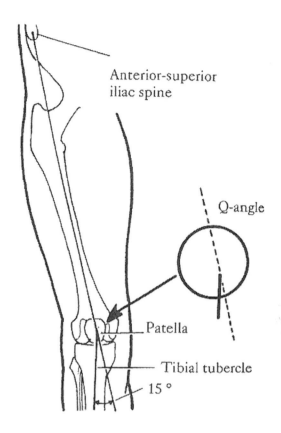

Anterior-superior
iliac spine

Q-angle

Patella

Tibial tubercle

15 °

The Q-angle is ideally 15 degrees. An angle greater than
20 degrees indicates increased risk of improper tracking
and perhaps chondromalacia. Because of wider hip bones,
women are at greater risk, as are athletes who overdevelop
quadriceps muscles and put uneven strain on the kneecap.

Symptoms

Initially, vague pain occurs when the kneecap moves outside the
femoral groove. A grating or crunching accompanies knee bending. Pain
increases with strain on the kneecap—squatting, lunging, or downhill
walking. As the cartilage softens, swelling and tenderness spread from a
focus on the kneecap in particular to the knee in general.

Solutions

With chondromalacia, pressing on the kneecap causes pain.
Arthroscopy allows the physician to examine the back of the

kneecap for definite indications of weakening. Because the causes of
chondromalacia are mechanical and usually based on body structure,
no surgical intervention or miracle medicine can cure the condition;
however, a balanced exercise program including quadriceps exercises to
help reduce strain on the kneecap will help. Bicycling with the seat high
and the gears low provides good exercise. Anti-inflammatory drugs may
help relieve some inflammation caused by the misalignment.

Kneecap Dislocation
Problem

The ability to see the dislocated kneecap as a lump on the
side of the knee and the severe pain of the condition make kneecap
dislocation, or displacement, easily identifiable. It occurs in those who
have congenital knee deformities that make them prone to dislocation
(some can dislocate their kneecaps with their hands), and it happens
in patients with chondromalacia. Extreme stress on the kneecap can
force dislocation in any individual as the result of a sudden twisting
motion and quadriceps contraction. Kneecaps can be dislocated in car
accidents in which a driver's or passenger's kneecap smacks against
the dashboard when the person continues in motion after the car has
suddenly stopped.

Symptoms

Dislocation can be seen as well as felt. The knee will refuse to bear
weight and will respond to the displacement with intense pain.

Solutions

In knee dislocation, the kneecap will be noticeably out of place,
simply a bump on the side of the joint. Initially, in cases of dislocation,
a physician will use a splint or brace and design an exercise program to
strengthen the muscles holding the kneecap in place. If the kneecap is
dislocated more than three times, surgery may be required to stabilize
the knee.

Pain in the Sides of the Knee

Pain in the sides of the knee is characteristic of several conditions
involving structural problems. Iliotibial band friction syndrome,
sometimes referred to as "runner's knee," is focused on the outer area
of the knee. When damage occurs to a ligament, the question may be
less where the pain is (it is everywhere or, with nerve damage, nowhere)
and more where the instability is. Instability and pain may occur

predominantly on the outside (what physicians call the *lateral* aspect) or inside (*medial* aspect) of the knee.

Runner's Knee
Problem

Runner's knee, a general term for what doctors call *iliotibial band friction syndrome,* is a tendonitis or an irritation on the outside part of the knee. Physicians prefer the technical term because "runner's knee" is a term used to refer to any knee pain. The tensor fasciae latae muscle on the outside of the hip connects to a thin but very strong structure called the iliotibial band. This band then attaches to the bump on the outside of the knee and below the knee. When the knee extends and flexes, this band moves across the bony contour of the knee and becomes irritated. Cumulative irritation eventually causes pain. The friction may also irritate a small bursa underneath this attachment, causing localized bursitis here also.

Symptoms

The pain caused by this friction is very insidious. Many times when patients evaluate their activities, they find they have put more stress on this area than usual; for example, they have taken a longer-than-usual bike ride, run on the side of the road instead of on a track, or have taken long hikes after training with only short walks. Symptoms can vary from hurting all the time to only starting to hurt after so many times or after so many minutes into an activity. This pain is very unlikely to occur after participation in such non-weight-bearing sports as swimming.

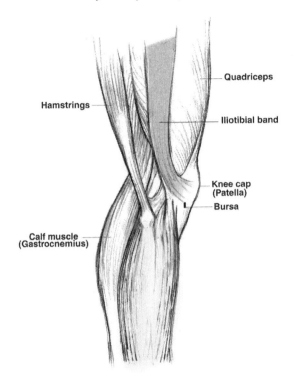

The iliotibial band connects hip muscles to the knee. Knee movement can cause the band to become irritated and result in pain on the outside of the knee.

Solutions

A common mistake in treatment is only treating where it hurts. Usually the pain is caused from tightness in the whole tensor fasciae latae muscle and iliotibial tract structure. Remember, the structure goes from the hip all the way to the knees; therefore, special types of stretches, such as Ober stretches, are used to stretch out the whole length and thus remove tension from the distal, or end, attachment. Deep tissue massage throughout the whole side of the leg is helpful, as are anti-inflammatory medicines. Occasionally a localized cortisone injection, treatment with cortisone pads, or localized electrical treatment may be beneficial. Sometimes the increased stress may be coming from misalignment of the knee or ankle, and exercises that are arthrotic may be beneficial.

Ligament Injury
Problem

The four main ligaments of the knee are the anterior and posterior cruciate ligaments and the medial and lateral collateral ligaments. The anterior cruciate (*cruciate* means "cross") is the front cross ligament of the knee. It prevents the tibia, or lower leg bone, from coming forward. Injury to this ligament is so common that *Sports Illustrated* once devoted an entire article to this ligament.

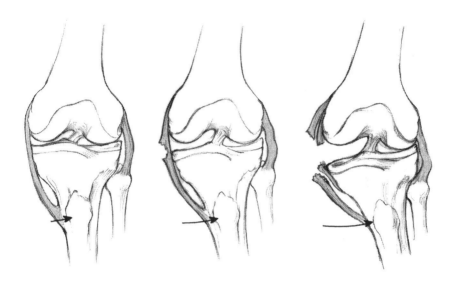

A first-degree sprain (left) causes tenderness and pain, but ligament function is unchanged. With a second-degree sprain (center), joint laxity is present along with pain. A third-degree sprain (right) brings dramatic instability and complete disruption to ligament function. Pain with a third-degree sprain may be less than in others because nerves may be severed, making pain intensity an unreliable guide to ligament damage.

The posterior cruciate ligament is the strongest ligament in the knee. It runs opposite to the anterior cruciate ligament and prevents the shinbone from going backward. Since it is so strong, it takes a much stronger blow to tear this ligament. The medial and collateral ligaments are on the sides of the knee. They are long, flat bands that prevent the limbs from becoming too knock-kneed or too bowlegged. We call these ligaments *varis* and *valgus,* respectively. If an athlete gets hit on the outside of the knee, it puts stress and pressure on the medial, or inside, collateral ligament. The opposite stress would cause injury or stress to the lateral collateral ligament. Ligament sprains are measured in degrees. Imagine your interlocked fingers as the ligament, and a first-degree sprain can be likened to pulling flatly and having your fingers stay in place. The length of the ligament fibers has not changed, but there is some injury, if only microscopic. A second-degree tear would be similar to pulling your interlocked fingers apart a bit. A slight lengthening of the ligaments results in some loosening of the joint in the direction the ligament protects. A third-degree injury would be similar to pulling your hands completely apart. Your fingers (the ligament fibers) would then be disconnected and a complete tear would exist. The degree of pain and swelling usually increases as the grade increases; however, in a complete, third-degree tear of the ligament, the pain fibers are also torn. Since they are torn or disconnected, many times this tear does not hurt as much as when the pain fibers are only stretched, as in the first- and second-degree injuries. For this reason, pain cannot be the sole guide to how badly a ligament is torn.

Ligaments can be strained by a traumatic or definite event or a chronic overload. In a traumatic injury, for example, the skier's tip gets caught, the binding does not release, and the knee goes inward. The ligament on the medial side of the knee (the medial collateral ligament) then sustains an immediate injury. A chronic overload would be caused by a person who is flatfooted and knock-kneed and goes running. Day after day there is increased stress on that ligament because of imbalance of alignment. Eventually stretching of the ligament and pain result because of chronic overload. Thus the mechanisms of injury can be very different.

Ligament strains can happen at work (when the floor is uneven and your foot falls into an unexpected depression) or on the sports field—especially in football, soccer, or rugby.

Symptoms

Pain is the foremost symptom of ligament strain and may vary from severe to excruciating. The knee will feel unstable and, if untreated, may be identified as a "trick" knee. A snap or an audible *pop* may accompany the injury. Afterward, if the pain disappears, it does not mean that all is well. It may mean that the nerves have also been damaged. When swelling immediately follows the injury, it indicates that blood has flowed into the joint, a natural consequence of the ligament's being ruptured or torn. The damage can vary from a slight overstretching to a complete rupture, detaching the ligament from the thighbone above it or from the shinbone below it. If you hear a *pop* and the telltale swelling follows within four hours, ice your knee, take acetaminophen (Tylenol)—not aspirin (it will facilitate bleeding)—and see a doctor.

Injuries to the separate ligaments produce different symptoms. When the collateral ligament is injured, patients usually describe a definite blow or twist and resulting pain along the ligament's course. If the anterior posterior ligament is injured, the pain, sometimes overwhelming, will be deep inside the knee. When this ligament is torn, though, pain may be absent or minimal if other ligaments are not injured. Injury to the anterior cruciate ligament produces blood inside the knee and swelling within 24 hours in 70% of cases. Therefore, immediate swelling after a knee injury is an ominous sign that there may be ligament damage. When the posterior cruciate ligament is injured, it often bleeds in the back of the knee, and the blood does not pool within the joint.

Solutions

Injury to a ligament requires immediate attention from a physician, who will determine the extent of the trauma and the scope of treatment. A sprain may require a splint or cast to immobilize the knee for three to six weeks. More severe injuries may require more dramatic treatment, such as surgery. A physician may decide to use arthroscopy to evaluate the injury and to determine the best course for restoring stability to the knee.

Exercises for strengthening the muscles may be an integral part of the rehabilitation process. Swimming, for example, is an excellent means of regaining functionality because it helps strengthen the muscles and restore stability without the strain of gravity.

If the ligaments fail to regain their strength, a brace designed for activity may be necessary if the patient wishes to continue sports known to produce these kinds of injuries. These specially made braces encircle the calf and the thigh, and they support the knee's top, bottom, and sides.

Meniscus Tear
Problem

The menisci, crescent-shaped fibrous cartilage between the shinbone and thighbone, are the shock absorbers of the knee. There are two in each knee, riding along each side of the knee like shock absorbers on a car. Like ligaments, they can be injured with severe twisting or jarring, weight-bearing movement. But unlike ligament injuries, meniscal injuries are not typically the result of traumatic events. They come from chronic stress. Repeated squatting or deep knee bends performed while putting pots and pans away in the kitchen, repairing a low fence or gate, or trying to get back in shape can cause the cartilage to separate horizontally or vertically. A torn fragment may be pushed into the inner knee, where it is crushed between the shinbone and thighbone. These injuries occur more frequently in men than in women, and more often in the medial meniscus (the one in the inner knee) than in the lateral (outer) one. Though not simple cartilage, the menisci are what people are usually referring to when they say someone suffered "torn cartilage in the knee."

Symptoms

Pain caused by the tear itself or the crushing of the fragment between the shinbone and thighbone usually is enough to send the injured looking for a physician. Pain from menisci tears differs from that of ligament sprains in that the knee will be tender along the joint line between the shinbone and thighbone on the side of the injured meniscus. The knee may lock, release, and then lock again because of the loose fragment interfering with normal motion. The knee may even click audibly.

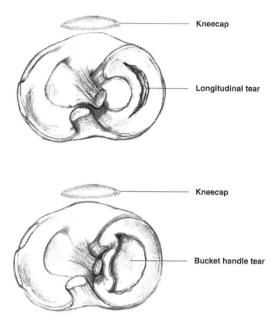

Kneecap

Longitudinal tear

Kneecap

Bucket handle tear

The menisci are crescent-shaped shock absorbers within the knee that are typically injured by repetitive stress rather than a traumatic injury. With repeated abuse, tears (top) advance to more dramatic conditions (bottom). Surgery to remove these disks is the seventh most commonly performed surgical procedure in the United States. A cutaway view of the knee (bottom) shows an intact meniscus on the right and a meniscus with a bucket handle tear on the left.

Solutions

Soreness at the joint line often helps the physician tell the difference between ligament and meniscal injuries. Repair, if the tear is clean, provides the best prospect for long-term mobility, but the four months required for recovery is considered by some a high price to pay. Repair is superior to menisectomy—total removal of the meniscus—because those who underwent menisectomy in their twenties found themselves with arthritis in the knee in their late forties, a much younger age than usual for onset of arthritis. Nonetheless, menisectomy is the seventh most commonly performed operation in the United States. Ironically, if the meniscus is removed, recovery is rapid, and if you are an athlete, you may be back to your workouts in three weeks.

Partial menisectomy is also an option, and a much better solution than total removal. Often the part of the meniscus that tears is the part that bears only about 30 percent of the weight. It can be trimmed away if it cannot be repaired, and the recovery period will be about the same as for a menisectomy.

Meniscal replacements and transplants, though performed, are still experimental. No one knows what the long-term results will be.

Synovial Tissue Overgrowth and Irritation
Problem

Almost everyone has synovial folds, or plicae, in their knees. The most common location is along the inner knee. Occasionally, a fold may be present above the kneecap. Ordinarily, the synovium lines the joint cavities of the knee, but sometimes an overgrowth of normal tissue occurs. These plicae usually dissolve; however, sometimes they partition and a remnant remains. If a patient performs an activity repetitively or suffers an injury to this area, the plica may become irritated. Once it becomes irritated, it gets larger. When it gets larger, it then can cause more mechanical problems, and a vicious cycle ensues.

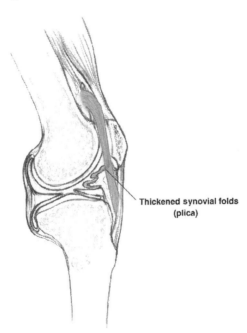

Thickened synovial folds
(plica)

A thickening of a synovial fold (plica) in the knee can become irritated by use and then worsen with more use.

Symptoms

The most common complaint is an aching on the inner side of the knee. If this plica is above the kneecap, some of the aching may be on the top of the knee. Usually patients complain of a feeling of tightness, and occasionally patients describe throbbing. The examiner may feel a plica popping across the femoral cartilage or bone as the knee extends or bends. This symptom is most commonly seen in patients who participate in sports in which running is integral. This condition should not be confused with chondromalacia, or roughening underneath the kneecap, or a medial cartilage tear. In an adolescent, the pain is usually a plica or possibly kneecap pain as opposed to frank wearing or chondromalacia of the kneecap. Only relatively few people have a plica requiring treatment.

Solutions

Treatment essentially consists of rest, anti-inflammatory medicines, and ice when the knee is acutely irritated. The condition requires giving attention to alignment of the knee and ankle, and the patient may have to modify activity for a short time. Oral anti-inflammatory drugs are usually helpful, and occasionally a cortisone shot into the plica area is necessary. A neoprene brace can be of benefit. When all conservative measures have failed and diagnostic imaging by X-ray and magnetic resonance imaging does not show any kneecap problem or meniscal problem, the patient may be a candidate for arthroscopic surgery. This operation is very successful if indeed the patient has a pathologic plica.

Loose Bone or Cartilage within the Knee
Problem

Loose pieces of bone or cartilage, called "joint mice" or "loose bodies," may float suspended in the knee's synovial fluid without causing discomfort until they grow larger.

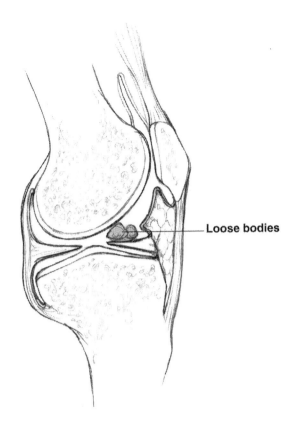

Loose bodies

Pieces of bone or cartilage sometimes float suspended within the knee's natural fluid, only causing pain when they grow large. They can cause knees to lock or grind on movement.

Symptoms

Beginning small and producing only a simple muted *snap* or *crackle,* joint mice cause trouble only when they interfere with normal motion, resulting in grinding or locking of the knee.

Solutions

X-ray films or magnetic resonance imaging films are the best means of visualizing joint mice from torn cartilage. Arthroscopic removal of the loose body is the typical solution, but sometimes open, or traditional, surgery is required. Recovery following arthroscopic removal lasts about three weeks.

Local Arthritis
Problem

Local arthritis is a condition that is very rapid in onset. Physicians give it a long name—*localized spontaneous osteonecrosis*—and like any arthritis of the joint, the condition is characterized by inflammation (*osteo* means "bone" and *necrosis* means "dying"). The bone in a localized area dies somehow, possibly because of losing its blood supply. The patients are usually sixty or more years of age, but it can occur in patients in their forties. The exact mechanism or cause of this condition remains unidentified.

Symptoms

Patients usually describe a very definite onset of pain. It is not usually associated with trauma or with twisting the knee. The pain is usually medial (the part of the knee touching the other knee) or on the inside of the knee. Patients feel like their knee gives way or locks. Upon further questioning, the patient does not report a definite unlocking of the knee but rather a gradual return of motion. Swelling is sometimes associated with this. The diagnosis is usually made by X-ray films, although they are commonly normal initially. A computerized tomography scan or magnetic resonance image of the bone may be useful.

Solutions

The initial treatment is supportive with anti-inflammatory medicines, crutches, rest, and exercises. These localized areas can sometimes heal over the next few months; however, many times, particularly if the necrosis can be seen on an X-ray, the lesions will worsen and the patient's problems will persist. If the area remains localized, either a bony realignment of the knee, a replacement of the cartilage where the osteonecrosis is located, or a total knee replacement may be necessary, depending on the person's age. The older the person, the more likely a knee replacement will be required.

Pain in the Front or Back of the Knee

Tendonitis and hamstring strain, representing respectively pain in the front and the back of the knee, are familiar opponents of weekend warriors, those ambitious adults whose work weeks are packed with over sedentary work and whose weekends are packed with—well, you guessed it—overactive play. Even if sometimes the "play" is the work of keeping up the home and yard—gardening, lawn tending, home repairing. These injuries that result from overuse can seem mild but pack a painful punch with time.

Tendonitis
Problem

Tendons, cords, or tissue that connect muscles to the bone, transfer the action of the muscle to it. But when tendons are overused, they respond with inflammation. Pain, redness, and swelling occur. This tendonitis, or inflammation of the tendons, usually results from overuse. Too much stress on a poorly conditioned tendon may be the culprit.

Tendonitis can be acute (coming on quickly and lasting only briefly) or chronic (recurring repetitively). Gymnasts who practice a hard landing over and over again during one three-hour training session might get acute tendonitis in their kneecap. Basketball players and volleyball players get this same kind of tendonitis and call it "jumper's knee." Runners who dramatically increase their training for an upcoming marathon may get tendonitis on the outside of their knee, in what is called the *iliotibial tract*.

Symptoms

Tendonitis, unlike many other knee injuries, allows an athlete to continue using the leg. Though it may hurt when initiating the activity, the pain may disappear after the first 15 minutes or so of warm-up. The pain won't return until the next day when it will be worse. Tendonitis, very forgiving in the beginning, becomes more severe with repeated infractions. With acute tendonitis, an athlete can continue to use the knee, but ignoring the grating or sandy feeling when the tendon moves through its sheath may permit the tendonitis to become a chronic condition.

Solutions

To help prevent tendonitis and other injuries, always stretch thoroughly before working out. Slow and gradual stretches, without bouncing, that are held for at least six seconds get the blood moving and help accustom the body to movement. Acute knee tendonitis requires RICE (rest, ice, compression, and elevation). When the swelling goes down, change the therapy: apply heat before workouts and ice afterward. Until the injury heals, take aspirin or another anti-inflammatory drug. Revise your workouts to be kind to your knees for at least two weeks.

Chronic tendonitis needs heat or contrast therapy, the alternating of 5-minute heat and 5-minute ice compresses totaling 20 minutes, and massage. In contrast therapy, heat improves circulation and thereby healing and the ice reduces or controls the swelling from the increased circulation. But chronic tendonitis, like acute tendonitis, once healed, is best followed by a muscle exercise program so that the system can be made stronger and a recurrence prevented.

Hamstring Strain
Problem

The hamstrings, or muscles along the back of the thigh, extend the hip joint and flex the knee joint. They smooth the movement of these joints, but they rebel from performing their duties when an unusual load is placed on them. Then they are torn instead of being normally stretched. This rebellion is most likely to occur when workouts have been prolonged and muscles, because they are tired, have lost their elasticity. In a defiant "No!" the hamstring contracts in a spasm, a natural defense against more strain.

Symptoms

An athlete may feel the hamstring sprain anywhere from the ischial tuberosity of the pelvis (the bones on which he sits) to the attachment at the upper tibia. These sprains happen suddenly and the resultant pain feels like the aftereffects of a swift kick.

The natural contraction resulting from hamstring sprain limits the scope of movement. But range of movement is relative. Such a strain can prevent a person who can usually touch her toes from being able to do it. A gymnast I treated was able to bring her left foot behind her and practically over her head, but I sensed that her hamstring was nonetheless strained. Why? Because when I asked her to perform the same action with her right leg, she was able to take her right foot well over the top of her head. Hamstring strain was limiting what was for her usual scope of movement.

Solutions

Immediately applying ice anesthetizes the area, and slowly stretching the muscle will help relieve the spasm. Heavy pressure maintained at the focus of the pain is an alternative to stretching. If these methods fail, a muscle relaxant may be required. Aspirin or ibuprofen will help prevent inflammation.

When the initial shock and pain have receded, keep the muscle warm and take pressure off of it by wrapping it in a neoprene pant or an elastic bandage in a figure eight. The torn muscle needs time to recuperate. Though painful, hamstring strains are relatively common, and even if the muscle is seriously ruptured, the necessity of surgical repair is highly unlikely.

Growth Plate Inflammation
Problem

Occurring most commonly in fourteen- to sixteen-year-olds who are athletic, growth plate inflammation (Osgood-Schlatter disease) is characterized by warmth, reddening, and pain on the growth plate at the top front part of the shinbone where the kneecap tendon attaches to hold the kneecap in place. The growth plate (the tibial tuberosity) is weak and irritated because of growth and activity. Though the cause of growth plate inflammation is not known, physicians theorize that it occurs because weak quadriceps muscles allow too much force to be transmitted to the growth plate through the tendon from the quadriceps.

Symptoms

This condition produces an achy knee, in which pain centers on the front at the "bump." Running or playing sports brings severe pain.

Solutions

Rest, ice, and elevation are the usual recommendations for mild cases. If an activity hurts, don't do it. Decreasing running distance or time spent at an activity may be enough, or refraining completely from athletic activity may be necessary. Splints may be recommended by some physicians. As growth decreases, the risk of Osgood-Schlatter disease decreases. When the growth plate fuses and the bone solidifies, the risk disappears. In mild cases, improving quadriceps strength will help.

Patellar-Femoral Syndrome
Problem

Pain in the front of the knee between the kneecap and thighbone is commonly seen in adolescents and young adults. The crunching or grating that patients feel and hear in their knees is a result of significant wearing. The kneecap normally glides in a well-aligned groove, and if this does not occur or there is some kind of abnormality in the cartilage, pain may ensue. Patients may feel pain without any direct wearing of the cartilage, or the wearing may progress all the way through the cartilage into the bone. This condition can be quite problematic because as long as you have a kneecap there is potential for irritation.

Patellar-femoral syndrome may be a temporary condition caused by doing an activity one is not used to, for example, riding a bike for an extended time or with the seat too low. Vigorous knee extension exercises on a knee machine may also cause this. Sometimes running is the cause, if there is not good alignment in the foot (overpronation) or there is not good alignment of the knee, whether the patient is bowlegged or knock-kneed. Experts also think some metabolic abnormality in the cartilage can cause pain in this area.

Symptoms

Patients are many times embarrassed because they cannot specifically locate the pain. They point to areas all around the kneecap and deep in the knee. This is because the kneecap is a large round structure in the front of the knee and can circumferentially radiate pain. Pain is usually worse when arising from a sitting position and going down inclines or stairs. That's because going down actually loads the knee more than going up. Many times patients will complain of the knee's popping or grating.

Solutions

Exercises and modifying activity are mainstay treatments for this kneecap-thighbone pain. Initially, ice, rest, and anti-inflammatory drugs calm the irritation. This axiom is applicable to almost any inflammatory process. Then the physician must look at causes: alignment, shoe wear, poor bracing or support (orthotics), and muscle strength. Many times, the patient has either gained weight or been less active and thus started the vicious cycle of weakness and pain. Neoprene supports are helpful. If the patient is a runner, she may be encouraged to continue her activities but to do them in a non-weight-bearing sense, by doing aqua jogging or biking with the seat high. It may be surprising that the stair-stepping kind of exercise seems to be well-tolerated. This is because the leg muscles are strengthened without the shock of running and jumping.

Summary

About half of all Americans participate in sports, and about the same percentage of adult Americans have experienced a knee injury sometime during their life. Others have injured their knees by simply doing their jobs or hurt their knees with an overly zealous weekend agenda of painting or gardening or running. Without a hinge to hold them in place, the parts of the knee work in a miracle of interplay of give and take. And its miraculous construction sees the knee through considerable abuse. Conditioning and stretching before working out go a long way toward preventing injuries, as will listening to your body (see Chapter 2). When injuries strike, be ready with the therapies recommended here, including rest, ice, compression, and exercise, and be ready to consult a physician when swelling fails to subside, signs of infection such as redness appear, or fractures seem evident.

5

When You Have Arthritis

"For all the happiness mankind can gain / Is not in pleasure, but in rest from pain."
—John Dryden

*R*achel Carr, in her book Listen to Your Inner Self, *tells of her survival of unremitting pain and depression from arthritis that began in her teens. A spinal injury, supposedly the result of a childhood accident, caused spinal nerve pressure that was eventually diagnosed as osteoarthritis. Treatment with large doses of aspirin for symptomatic relief of pain caused internal bleeding. Treatment in her twenties encompassed traction that brought little relief and left her exhausted from long sleepless nights. Cortisone injections were attempted and then discontinued because of intolerance. "The pain spread with full force, paralyzing me at times," she wrote, admitting that her arthritis forced her to retreat to bed, which resulted in muscle degeneration and joint pain and stiffness. Every physician she consulted would take new X-rays and announce that the spinal calcification had increased.*

Finally, she turned to an Indian yogi, who encouraged her and gave her hope. His program for renewal called for recruiting the body's own healing powers to heal her. She followed his plan of physical exercise, deep breathing, and meditation, and these gradually pushed the chronic pain, swelling, and depression out of her life. They became the wellspring from which she drew renewal after assaults on her being. "To gain equanimity," she wrote, "we must unite the body with the mind so we can ride either on the crest or in the trough of waves with a steady hand at the helm. Isn't this what life is all about?"

Almost 43 million people in the United States suffer from arthritis. For them, poet John Dryden's words, written in the epigraph above, are achingly true. Not like a case of chicken pox or flu, arthritis is long lasting; and like cancer, arthritis is not one disease but many. More than

100 conditions are properly classified as types of arthritis, but all have different sets of symptoms, diagnostic tests, and patterns of treatment and care. Pain, though, is a common factor. It is no wonder arthritis sufferers feel overwhelmed at times.

Arthritis is the leading cause of disability in the United States, preventing millions from doing what others their age can do. Only heart disease outpaces arthritis as a cause of work disability. Arthritis is more common in women than in men, and it is more common in elders: almost one of every two Americans 65 years of age or older has it. This means, of course, that as the population ages, more and more people will have arthritis—60 million by 2020, according to estimates.

An "old" disease, arthritis appears unwilling to yield completely the secrets of its causes or cures. It is a disease that has been found in fossil remains of creatures that lived 100 million years ago and in the skeletons of ancient humans. Records of gout can be found in medieval manuscripts, but reports of rheumatoid arthritis were first recorded only about 200 years ago. Unlike other old diseases that generally seem to be on the decline, arthritis is increasing. Of those younger than 65 years who have arthritis, two million are permanently disabled, and their lost wages are thought to total $50 billion per year.

Characteristics That Increase Risk and Modifying Behavior to Reduce Risk

Certain characteristics increase the risk of having arthritis, but the most common one—increasing age—is not something that can be changed. Sex is another. Women are more prone than men to degenerative arthritis, lupus, and fibromyalgia (a type of rheumatism), and men are more likely than women to have ankylosing spondylitis. Twice as many women as men experience osteoarthritis of the knee. Repetitive use or overuse also puts an individual at increased risk, but in some careers, including carpet laying, house cleaning, or playing catcher in professional baseball, long-term occupational joint stress can only be modified, not eliminated. Being overweight also puts individuals, especially women, at increased risk of osteoarthritis of the knees. One report published in the prestigious British medical journal *Lancet* in 1998 stopped short of blaming high heels for some cases of osteoarthritis of the knee in women, choosing instead to say that "the altered forces at the knee caused by walking in high heels may predispose to degenerative changes."

Arthritis and Your Knees

Arthritis is inflammation of any joint, and it can be traced to infectious, metabolic, or constitutional causes in adults or to heredity in young people. Thus, came the term *arthr-* or *arthro—*, which is the Latin combining form meaning "joint," and—*itis,* indicating inflammation. One or more joints become painful, stiff, and less functional or nonfunctional. The Arthritis Foundation, the chief nonprofit U.S. organization dedicated to making arthritis better understood and better treated, recommends that professional help from a physician be sought whenever pain, swelling, or trouble moving a joint persists for more than two weeks. During that time, physicians recommend that patients relieve their pain with aspirin or ibuprofen.

Blood tests for arthritis are not always conclusive. Patients with rheumatoid arthritis may have normal results. X-ray examinations may show change or variations from normal, scoliosis, less joint space, spurs, or what physicians call *tophi. Tophi* are chalky deposits that form around joints and cause the body to respond as it does to any foreign invader—with inflammation. These deposits, made of sodium urate and characteristic of gout, may be found in tissue or bursae, those fluid-filled sacs meant to prevent friction near bone, as well as in cartilage or bone. Bone scans, magnetic resonance imaging, computerized tomography (CAT) scanning, and specialized types of blood tests may be required to accurately diagnose a condition.

Gout and joint infections are considered types of arthritis, but rheumatoid arthritis and osteoarthritis are the types most familiar to most people. Twice as many people are affected by rheumatoid arthritis as are affected by gout, and osteoarthritis affects about five times as many people as are affected by those two combined (see figure). Osteoarthritis is the type of arthritis that most often affects knees. Characterized by the gradual wearing away of cartilage, knee osteoarthritis usually results from the wear and tear of bearing a load over time. Other parts of the knee, including ligaments, muscles, and tendons, may also be affected. Coping remains an important element in managing life after diagnosis with the disease.

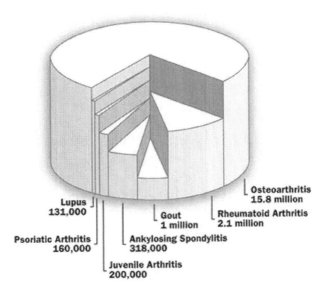

Osteoarthritis is the most common type of arthritis, and it is the type that most commonly affects knees. Rheumatoid arthritis and pseudogout (an arthritic condition that mimics gout and is more often found in the knees than gout) also affect the knee joint. These are estimates for common forms of arthritis. (Reprinted from C. J. Strange, "Coping with Arthritis in Its Many Forms," a revised version of an article published in FDA Consumer [1996] and retrieved from *http://www.fda.gov/fdac/graphics/1996graphics/arthritis. jpeg*).

Research shows that outcome from arthritis depends at least as much on the patient's own actions as on treatments. Physicians who understand how patients feel about their arthritis are probably more likely to be able to help them. Weiner and Goss in *The Complete Book of Homeopathy* (Avery Publishing Group, 1989) suggest that too often the approach is to suppress the symptoms with drugs without identifying the underlying causes, thereby allowing the disease itself to progress. People with arthritis have difficulty with daily activities, and emotional problems can cause or exacerbate arthritis. People who have better coping abilities do better with arthritis. Mike and Nancy Samuels, in their book *Arthritis: How to Work with Your Doctor and Take Charge of Your Health,* describe Aaron Antonovsky's theory about patients' ability to cope with illness. Antonovsky argues that seeing problems that arise as opportunities and not threats is part of a health-promoting world view. Part of seeing the world this way is believing that the world is comprehensible, believing that one can cope or manage life and its changes whether alone or with help, and believing that life has meaning and is worth emotional investment. People who have these beliefs cope better with arthritis—and with other challenges of life. Arthritis also tends to be better tolerated by people who have more than twelve years of education. Arthritis is compounded in patients who have experienced long-term tension and anger in their lives.

This chapter will examine three of the most common types of arthritis that attack the knee—osteoarthritis, rheumatoid arthritis, and pseudogout—and then discuss coping mechanisms.

Osteoarthritis

The most common form of arthritis, osteoarthritis, is what happens when the wear and tear on our bones surpasses our body's ability to repair the cartilage that protects it, and bone begins to rub against bone. Like metal rubbing against metal in the absence of a gasket or like glass hitting glass when the rubber seal is missing on an airtight jar, bone grates against bone in arthritis causing pain. Osteoarthritis can occur without evident cause (primary idiopathic osteoarthritis), or it can result from injury to a joint (secondary osteoarthritis). A joint can be injured by a fracture, an infection inside it, damage by disease (gout or diabetes), or other cause. It can strike as early as the teenage years, and by the time people reach their forties, 90 percent of them have experienced the changes in their cartilage from which osteoarthritis arises. For only one of five, though, the changes that usually occur over many years have been dramatic enough to send them to a doctor who diagnoses their problem as osteoarthritis. In fact, X-ray films can show evidence of osteoarthritis that has caused the patient no problems or pain.

For many, osteoarthritis begins in their knees. The hands are the next most likely target and hips follow. Men are more likely than women to discover it in the spine. Activity, including overuse of joints, is often associated with these changes, as is carrying heavy loads, including too much body weight. Because knees must carry a load on bending of four to eight times a person's weight (a load manageable when the person is of average weight), obese individuals often find the pain in their knees is caused by osteoarthritis. A diet high in saturated fats or a low-activity lifestyle may also contribute to the problem. Coal miners who must carry heavy weights have osteoarthritis in their hips and knees. Pain is typically greatest after exercise or joint use, but it may fade in the early stages of osteoarthritis. With time, pain may linger after joint use or may even cause sleeplessness at night. Joints may swell or not and may be warm to the touch.

As osteoarthritis progresses, the patient may be able to hear the bones actually rubbing against each other. Called *crepitus,* this announcement to all that the joint is no longer cushioned the way it used to be can be embarrassing as well as disconcerting. *Osteophytes,* extensions of the bone that appear as hard lumps along joint edges or margins, cause pain on touch and by injuring nerves. Bone spurs are typical of these abnormal growths. Though most people learn to live with their osteoarthritis over time, about 25 percent experience progressive crippling and increasing pain that reduces function and proves destabilizing.

A physician makes a diagnosis of osteoarthritis by measuring sedimentation rate of erythrocytes, which may be normal or slightly elevated, and by having the patient get an X-ray of the joint. X-rays can reveal a narrowing of the space between the joints, wearing of the bone, osteophytes forming on the bone margins, and possibly bone cysts. To rule out rheumatoid arthritis, the physician may screen the blood for rheumatoid factor. A physician may take a sample of the synovial fluid out of the affected joint and have it analyzed to classify the case properly as noninflammatory (characteristic of osteoarthritis), inflammatory (characteristic of rheumatoid or psoriatic arthritis, or gout), or septic (characteristic of a bacterial infection).

Treatment for Osteoarthritis of the Knee

Treatment for osteoarthritis of the knee aims to relieve pain and prevent disability. Drugs used for the treatment of osteoarthritis include aspirin and other pharmaceuticals called nonsteroidal anti-inflammatory drugs (NSAIDs). They are nonsteroidal, which means they are not steroids, a class of molecules that plays a variety of parts in living things. Steroids, such as hormones, regulate cell activity throughout the body. They are powerful because once the steroid hormone connects with a receptor within a target cell, the complex they create can cause fundamental changes in the cell's biology.

NSAIDs include those that are salicylates and those that are nonsalicylates. Examples of salicylates include aspirin (acetylsalicylate), magnesium and choline salicylate. Nonsalicylates include fenoprofen calcium (Nalfon), naproxen (Naprosyn), ibuprofin (Motrin), indomethacin (Indocin), meloxicam (Mobic), tolmetin (Tolectin), sulindac (Clinoril), and celecoxib (Celebrex), to name a few. Because individuals respond differently to each drug, a patient may find relief with one NSAID but not another. Other drugs obtainable without a prescription include nontraditional, or alternative, remedies such as glucosamine sulfate and chondroitin. Another is an analgesic cream that contains capsaicin, the chemical in hot peppers responsible for their heat. It has proven to be a helpful over-the-counter remedy for those suffering from osteoarthritis. To avoid getting the capsaicin in the eyes, nose, or other sensitive body area, wash your hands carefully after applying the cream.

Abide by these rules when taking NSAIDs or other nonprescription remedies to combat osteoarthritis:

- Use the lowest dose that proves effective, and use it for the shortest time possible.
- Take drugs with food.
- Tell your doctor what you are taking.
- Never substitute a self-prescribed medicine for one prescribed for you by your physician.
- Consult your physician before mixing prescription drugs with over-the-counter medicines and alternative medicine therapies in any combination.

The nutritional supplements glucosamine sulfate and chondroitin, made from animal products, have been widely reported to benefit those suffering from osteoarthritis. While many patients have embraced these dietary supplements, some physicians have remained skeptical. They believe the results of the studies were not reliable. Why? Because in some cases the supplements' manufacturers had paid for the studies and their employees participated in them. To investigate the merit of scientific studies backing the positive claims, four researchers from the Arthritis Center at Boston University School of Medicine performed an analysis of six glucosamine trials and nine chondroitin trials, all of which included patients with arthritis of the knee and all of which measured pain or functional outcome. Their findings were published in the *Journal of the American Medical Association* in March 2000, and they concluded that the products were probably effective to some degree. Other research continues.

A survey conducted by the Arthritis Foundation found that glucosamine was a favorite alternative therapy of almost 800 men and women with arthritis. Thirty four percent of those surveyed said they used it. Only prayer (53 percent), meditation (38 percent), and visualization (37 percent)—all nondrug therapies—ranked higher. Altogether, 51 percent of those surveyed reported being "somewhat" interested in alternative therapies, and 28 percent reported being "highly" interested. The top alternative therapy recommended by physicians interviewed by the Arthritis Foundation was capsaicin: 78 percent of 2,146 physicians interviewed endorsed it.

A widely sold prescription arthritis medicine is celecoxib, which is marketed as Celebrex. Called a "cox-2 inhibitor," celecoxib affects prostaglandin production by inhibiting cyclo-oxygenase-2 (cox-2), an enzyme. When uninhibited, cox-2 enzymes promote inflammation and pain. The difference between NSAIDs and celecoxib is that while NSAIDs inhibit both cox-1 and cox-2 enzymes, celecoxib inhibits only cox-2. That's important because, when NSAIDs inhibit cox-1, the enzyme fails to do its job, which is to form a protective lining in the gastrointestinal tract and leave arthritis sufferers vulnerable to digestive tract problems. According to its co-marketers, Pharmacia Corporation and Pfizer, Inc., Celebrex is the only cox-2—specific inhibitor approved by the U.S. Food and Drug Administration for both osteoarthritis and adult rheumatoid arthritis. Worldwide, more than 21.5 million patients use the drug.

In clinical studies, celecoxib proved as effective in relieving pain and inflammation in patients with knee osteoarthritis and in patients with rheumatoid arthritis. Furthermore, it was associated with fewer instances of digestive tract ulcers and complications than were NSAIDs. Celecoxib may have other benefits, too. The National Cancer Institute is conducting studies to determine if celecoxib's ability to curb inflammation can help patients prone to colon cancer reduce their risk of the disease. Most cases of colon cancer develop from inflamed adenomatous polyps in the colon. It is also supporting research using celecoxib to treat other precancerous and cancerous conditions. However, note that it is always advisable to use caution with anti-inflammatory drugs. Vioxx (another cox-2 inhibitor) was recently taken off the market due to adverse cardiovascular problems.

As another solution to alleviate knee pain from osteoarthritis when pain medication fails, rheumatologists and orthopedic surgeons also inject a fluid into the knee that mimics the hyaluronic acid normally found in joint fluid. Supartz, Hyalgan, Synvisc, or Orthovisc, when injected three or more times, can bring relief for months.

Additionally, emerging technologies offer new hope for patients suffering from chronic conditions such as arthritis, osteoporosis, and tendon diseases. For example, Nuclear Magnetic Resonance Therapy (NMRT), which has been approved and used in Europe since 1999, can treat all stages of arthritis in all joints. This therapy was developed directly from Magnetic Resonance Imaging which, up until now, has been the most sophisticated and most expensive available diagnostic procedure. However, while conventional magnetic therapy uses only one axis, NMRT uses a three-dimensional magnetic field to directly superimpose resonant frequency on the carrier, exciting protons in damaged bone and cartilage cells and effectively reduces the symptoms of disease by growing cartilage in arthritic patients and increasing bone density for osteoporosis. Moreover, NMRT allows for custom therapy, enabling physicians to adjust the amount of the therapy depending on the particular needs of each individual patient. Studies of patients treated with NMRT have shown a marked increase in mobility and decrease in pain immediately following therapy. These figures dramatically improve during the first twelve months after the therapy. Apart from its effectiveness, NMRT is an attractive option because it involves no medication, is non-invasive, and has no known side effects. Additionally, the therapy is quite short. The patient receives treatment one hour per day on consecutive days, with the total therapy time ranging from three to ten hours.

Other remedies for knee osteoarthritis include bracing (which some patients find intolerable) and various surgical procedures that may be recommended based on many factors, including the age of the patient, his or her activity level, and specific characteristics of the case.

Exercise in Osteoarthritis

Because most patients with osteoarthritis have symptoms that never disappear but discomfort that only occasionally becomes incapacitating illness, the best advice is to keep moving. Since all exercise programs have to be individualized, patients must talk with their physicians or physical therapists to understand how to balance rest, especially when arthritis flares, with activity. Understandably, sometimes it is easier for arthritis sufferers to see what they cannot do rather than what they can do, but each one should try to find a type of exercise that will keep joints functioning and maintain range of motion. Swimming or biking or any activity that promotes exercise without forcing the joint to bear weight during the exercise is excellent for maintaining joint movement, not to mention improving outlook and energy level. The same reasons for exercising at any time—to increase flexibility, to improve strength and endurance, to increase range of motion, to improve circulation, to improve cardiovascular function—apply for undertaking an exercise program when arthritis is present. These activities include:

- biking, swimming, aqua jogging ("running" in a pool), low or no impact aerobics
- walking on a treadmill that includes working upper-body muscles against resistance
- rowing in a seated rower
- yoga

Patients who want to take it one step at a time may best separate their exercising into categories that indicate what their goal is (see exercises below). A basic goal might be to maintain range of motion and joint function. After succeeding at that goal, a patient might take on the harder task of strengthening muscles. After incorporating those kinds of exercises into a fitness routine, a patient could attempt aerobic exercise, important in maintaining or improving cardiovascular status. For most patients, the worst part of having arthritis is the fear that their illness could make them dependent on others. Exercising can help maintain function while improving mental outlook.

Exercises to Improve Range of Motion and Strength
Knees
- For Range of Motion Improvement:
- Pull knees toward you one at a time while lying on your back*
- With knees straight and legs extended, push knees down.

- For Strength Improvement:
- Lying flat on back, extend toes, pressing knees against surface, then pull toes in toward head.
- Sitting in a chair, slide one foot forward while simultaneously sliding the other back.

Fingers
- For Range of Motion Improvement:
- Draw each finger singly toward the thumb, creating a circle.
- Beginning with the thumb and the index finger forming a widely separated *V*, draw each finger singly toward the thumb.

- For Strength Improvement:
- With the palm flat on the table, try to move each finger toward the thumb with the fingertips of the other hand providing resistance.
- Place one hand on the table with palm down with the other on top with palm down. Try to raise and lower fingers one at a time with upper fingers providing resistance.

Hips

- For Range of Motion Improvement:
- While lying on back, move feet together and then far away from each other; or in same position with feet slightly apart, move feet inward and outward together.
- In erect position while resting pelvis against a counter or bar, lift leg backward and up with knee straight.

- For Strength Improvement:
- Add an elastic belt around ankles to the exercise in which legs are moved together and then far apart.
- Lift legs one at a time while lying on back. Keep knee of uplifted leg straight and knee of resting leg slightly bent.

Shoulders

- For Range of Motion Improvement:
- With fingers laced behind neck, move elbows in and out
- Holding a yardstick at either end with both hands, move stick over head.
- For Strength Improvement:
- Holding arms, encircled with elastic band, straight out in front, open arms against resistance of band.

Back

- For Range of Motion Improvement:
- With the feet flat on the floor and the knees bent, lie with back on the floor. Pull knees one at a time to chest.

NOTE: The function of certain exercises may overlap.

*This exercise also helps improve range of motion for hips and back.

Tips for Success with Exercising

- Make exercise a part of every day.
- Make an exercise plan based on recommendations from a physical therapist or a physician who knows you and your arthritis.
- Set realistic goals and accept progress, however slow.
- Schedule your exercises for a time when your medicine has its greatest effect.
- Take a hot bath or shower or use a hot pad on the affected joint immediately before beginning to exercise.
- Adjust the exercise program when it results in pain that lasts more than an hour.
- Balance exercising with rest.
- Try to continue to exercise gently during flares.

Rheumatoid Arthritis

Almost 90 percent of patients with rheumatoid arthritis report that their knees, usually both, are affected by the disease. It affects women two to four times more often than men, and with progression it can result in stiffness of the joint, deformity, and perhaps even loss of the ability to move about. That makes apparent that with rheumatoid arthritis, problems and complications are greater than with some other arthritic conditions.

The causes of rheumatoid arthritis are not known, but it is an autoimmune disease. For some reason, the body produces autoantibodies to an existing antigen, causing consequent injury to tissues. The sensitive synovial lining of the joint thickens and develops folds. Some scientists have speculated that a virus may cause the reaction. Archeologists have found no evidence in ancient skeletons of it, and no record of it exists before about 1800. Typically, a person suffers inflammation of corresponding joints in the arms or legs. Estimates for the percentage of the population affected range from one to four percent. Those most often affected are between 25 and 50 years of age, and most cases are characterized by chronic pain and an occasional attack of more serious symptoms.

Rheumatoid arthritis sufferers may experience early morning stiffness, pain, or tenderness at a joint or joints, swelling, and small nodules under the skin. They experience fatigue that is exacerbated by sleeplessness and eventually stiffness from inactivity. In a quarter of cases, the pain begins in a single joint, sometimes the knee. A person may gradually recognize a pattern to their collection of symptoms or, all of a sudden, the symptoms will descend in a dramatically brief period, perhaps even overnight, leaving the sufferer with fever, fatigue, and no appetite. For about 10 percent of patients, the first bout with rheumatoid arthritis is their one and only. Those who do not have rheumatoid arthritis until after they are 60 years old also are lucky— they typically experience a milder course than those who are diagnosed earlier.

Physicians use a blood test and X-rays to add further evidence to the diagnosis. They look for decalcification of the bones, particularly at the joints in question, being careful to differentiate degenerative changes from decalcification. In addition, they perform an agglutination test of the blood, looking for the rheumatoid factor. Other disorders affecting the joints have to be ruled out, such as systemic lupus erythmatosus, polyarteritis, progressive systemic sclerosis, sarcoidosis, or other disorders.

Treatment for Rheumatoid Arthritis of the Knee

Treatment for rheumatoid arthritis includes a combination of anti-inflammatory drugs, rest, and analgesics. Because aspirin taken in the high doses required for relief (a high dose might be 14 to 16 325-mg tablets daily) frequently causes gastrointestinal upset or even internal bleeding, physicians turn to NSAIDs as an alternative. NSAIDS usually recommended include fenoprofen calcium (Nalfon), naproxen (Naprosyn), ibuprofin (Motrin), indomethacin (Indocin), meloxicam (Mobic), tolmetin (Tolectin), sulindac (Clinoril), or celecoxib (Celebrex), although there are many others. If one doesn't work, then another may. A sufficient trial is necessary; it takes two to three weeks to determine effectiveness. Although these too can produce gastrointestinal upset and bleeding and have been associated with changes in the small intestine, they may be useful in supplementing the aspirin sufficiently to prevent adverse gastrointestinal effects.

Second-line therapies include methotrexate and gold. Methotrexate, a drug used in combination chemotherapy for cancer, was put to work on arthritis after dermatologists found that patients with psoriasis treated with methotrexate also reported improved arthritis. In studies of both children and adults, about 70 percent reported improvement. Women of child-bearing age need to protect against pregnancy while taking the drug, though, because a fetus can be affected by it. Other side effects include gastrointestinal intolerance, risk of liver damage, and adverse effects to bone marrow.

Gold has been a therapy for rheumatoid arthritis since the 1920s. Having fewer side effects than methotrexate, gold is an important second-line therapy. When administered by injection, gold is more effective but has more side effects than gold given orally.

Complementary therapies, other than those mentioned above, are acupuncture and herbalism. Acupuncture is a centuries-old Oriental technique used to restore the flow of *chi* throughout the body. Arthritis sufferers turn to acupuncture for relief of unrelenting pain. Studies of acupuncture give a mixed picture of its effectiveness. Anyone turning to an alternative therapy should understand the placebo effect and be ready to find objective measures as well as subjective ones to evaluate outcome. Foremost, those turning to acupuncture need to understand that acupuncture is an invasive procedure—the needles pierce the skin and should be of the disposable sort to ensure safety from infection.

Herbalists may recommend white willow bark as a painkiller. It contains the same chemical responsible for pain relief that is in aspirin. Useful, too, may be reviewing general nutrition. Perhaps a possible deficiency or eating habit may explain part of the lethargy or other characteristic that is part of the overall picture. Exercise increases muscle tone and improves outlook. People with arthritis who exercise feel like they are doing something to improve their well-being—and they are—when they exercise.

When medicine becomes inadequate to quell the pain and increasing disability imposed by rheumatoid arthritis, surgery may help. Options include synovectomy, in which a surgeon removes the joint lining (which regrows within a month). Undergoing the procedure may postpone recurrence for several years. As a last resort, patients with significant pain, evidence of joint destruction on X-ray, and other problems benefit from total knee replacement, regaining a high degree of movement with their knees.

Gout and Pseudogout

Gout arises when a metabolic failure results in injury to cartilage and joint. Hyperuricemia—too much uric acid in the blood—causes urate crystals to be deposited in and around the joints. They may appear in cartilage, bone, tissue beneath the skin, and even in the outer ear. When these crystals, or tophi, accumulate with advanced disease, they form lumps under the skin. The human system responds to these foreign bodies with inflammation, leaving joints swollen, red, and warm to the touch. Some patients cannot stand to have even a sheet touch the affected area. When these crystals continue to accumulate in the joint, where their insolubility in biologic fluids makes them difficult to remove, joints suffer erosive damage.

What causes the hyperuricemia are complications in the body's purine metabolism, abnormalities that can be genetic or acquired. The problem may be that too much uric acid is being produced by the body or that too little is being excreted by the kidneys. Hyperuricemia is sometimes found as one piece of a bigger medical picture. Ailments linked to gout are diseases affecting blood cell production, psoriasis, disorders of the thyroid gland, advanced kidney disease, and obesity.

Gout is characterized by a series of unexpected severe attacks of inflamed joints of the hands or legs and feet. Often gout strikes the big toe. What sets off these attacks may be excessive drinking or eating, stress, minor trauma, illness or surgery, or reaction to some drugs (e.g., insulin or penicillin), or some diuretics. During these attacks, pain increases progressively and dramatically and the skin over the joint may become red or purple, hot, and shiny. Initial rounds may be brief (three days or so), but without treatment, a patient's disease may become chronic, attacks will lengthen, and joint deformity will ensue.

In pseudogout, the mechanism of the arthritic condition is the same, but the crystals are made of a form of calcium, not uric acid. Having gout increases one's risk of having pseudogout, as do advanced osteoarthritis and joint disorders related to nerves. Whereas gout most often affects the big toe, pseudogout is more likely to affect the knee.

Men are much more likely to have gout than women, but they are no more likely than women to have pseudogout. Gout affects about a half million people, and most are between thirty and sixty years of age. Pseudogout most often affects those 70 years of age and older.

Diagnosing gout may be done simply by a physical examination and health history or by microscopic examination of crystals extracted from tophi or joint fluid. Physicians also look at a patient's response to colchicine, which usually produces relief within 48 hours. A patient with pseudogout will have evidence on X-rays of calcium deposits, often in the knee, and a milder set of symptoms. Identifying pseudogout definitively requires confirmation that the crystals extracted from joint fluid are made of calcium pyrophosphate dihydrate.

Treatment for Gout and Pseudogout

Once identified, gout can be treated effectively with drugs. NSAIDs, for example, ibuprofen or sulindac, can be used to moderate the inflammatory response and reduce the pain of the acute attacks. Whether the patient's problem is overproduction or retention of uric acid, specific drugs can be prescribed to prevent production or increase excretion. Efforts to reduce the risk of a gout attack will include watching weight and diet, and following recommendations of other physicians who are consulted.

Aspirin, because it may contribute to retaining uric acid in the blood, should not be taken. Acetaminophen (Tylenol), though a good pain reliever, has been surpassed by ibuprofen in inflammation-fighting properties. Drugs that may complicate gout include diuretics prescribed for weight loss or to lower blood pressure. These drugs slow clearance of uric acid from the body, putting patients at higher risk of a gout attack. Prednisone, a steroidal anti-inflammatory, may be used to treat gout, and colchicine, which physicians have used for centuries, still has a role in gout therapy. A physician should be consulted about changing any prescription medicine.

Modifying the diet can also soften the symptoms of gout. Foods high in purines (greater than 130 mg/3 ounces), such as kidney, liver, sweetbreads, and heart, should be avoided altogether, and those with greater than or equal to 50 mg purines per 3-ounce serving, such as lentils, spinach, and all fish, meat, and poultry, should be limited to one serving per day. Of alcoholic drinks, beer may be the most damaging because its purine level is higher than wine or other drinks. Some physicians warn patients to avoid all alcohol. Others suggest that if a person cannot resist it, alcohol should be blunted in effect by flushing the system with water (a good recommendation for general health) or by absorbing it with carbohydrates.

Therapy for pseudogout usually includes high doses of NSAIDs. As in gout, colchicine may relieve symptoms. Injecting steroids into the joint has proven to be beneficial to some patients, as has withdrawing joint fluid from the affected joint.

Coping with Arthritis

The profile of the situation of Rachel Carr presented at the beginning of this chapter is not unfamiliar territory to those who face chronic arthritis. Calling on her body's existing strengths and struggling to fortify every gain, she followed a program of physical exercise, deep breathing, and meditation, which brought relief and renewal.

Carr compares her method for deep breathing with the uptake of water by a flower. In other words, it should be slow, deep, and ultimately recognized as essential to life. Beginning with abdominal breathing that involves the diaphragm and abdomen as well as the lungs, she proposes moving forward to rib-cage breathing and to what she calls "complete" breathing. She advocates practicing abdominal breathing on the floor with knees bent, concentrating on the rise and fall of the abdomen and lengthening exhalation to twice the time of inhalation. For rib-cage breathing, she also recommends doubling the exhalation, suggesting that one inhale to the count of five and exhale to the count of 10. One may stand or sit erect, with hands on the rib cage, concentrating on the in and out movement of the rib cage and chest. The same pattern follows for complete breathing, but the focus here is on continuous, rhythmic breathing that is like pouring water into one vessel and then pouring it back into another.

Carr proposes a ten-week program meant to help patients cultivate the healing power within them. She endorses yoga and the depression-defeating rhythmic breathing and meditation. For Carr, China's theory of *chi* and India's theory of *prana* became ways of thinking about how to achieve balance of the body and mind. Breathing can involve the abdomen or the rib cage alone or it can incorporate moving both. Visualization can become a part of the process. You can put your hands on the area of pain or you can focus your mind on it. She imagines breathing out the negative energy and the pain associated with the arthritis. Breathing rhythmically, the patient can imagine that with the ebb and flow of breath the blood flows into the area and thoughts should focus on good things.

Carr integrates touch with deep breathing to harness healing energy and to focus it on a source of pain. Touching the area of pain is not necessary but may help in focusing. She says to visualize each inhalation as an absorption of healing energy and each exhalation as a release of pain, and to reject a focus on illness and to imagine wellness and strength. She advises repeating, "I will get better. I am better. I feel no pain. I am free of pain." Breathing rhythmically and focusing on the rise and fall of breathing are meant to bring relaxation and greater tranquility. Thinking good thoughts and imagining the flow of blood to the troubled site reinforce the benefits of the breathing.

This approach succeeded in another context in a personal experience. Once before surgery, I came into the surgical suite preoperatively to reassure the patient before the anesthesia took effect. He was there for knee surgery, and as I began to talk to him I placed my hand on his knee. "Doctor," he said to me, "I feel warmth and healing in your hand, in your touch." This fellow was a tough, burly guy, and I felt sure this kind of response was deeply felt and impulsively spoken, not a rehearsed reply spoken out of duty to some belief system or for effect.

In 1964 , author and editor, Norman Cousins, was diagnosed with ankylosing spondylitis, a degenerative arthritis characterized by the disintegration of connective tissue in the spine. At the time, spondylitis was treated with aspirin and phenylbutazone, drugs whose use Cousins questioned as being more toxic than therapeutic. He reasoned that aspirin was antagonistic to the body's ability to nurture and support the connective tissue whose failure was the cause of his illness. He gave it up, started taking vitamin C instead, and turned for pain relief to the anesthetic effects of laughter, induced in his case by old movie and television comedies. He improved. His sedimentation rate—the measure of the fall of red cells in a tube of drawn blood—dropped from a high indicating serious inflammation to levels, though not dramatically lower, that were indicative of cumulative improvement. The response was characterized as "the placebo effect": he improved because he believed he would.

Cousins also describes the placebo effect at work in other cultures. The author had visited Dr. Alfred Schweitzer, the famed physician of the twentieth century who was a humanitarian and doctor in Lambaréné, West Gabon, a country on Africa's western coast. After Cousins remarked that the Africans were certainly much better off in Dr. Schweitzer's care than in the care of African witch doctors, Schweitzer arranged a visit to a witch doctor's practice. After observing patient—witch doctor interaction for a couple of hours, Schweitzer explained what they had observed on their return to his clinic. He said that the witch doctor's patients fell into three categories: those with functional complaints, which he treated by supplying the patients with herbs; a second group had ailments generally psychogenic in nature, which the witch doctor treated with incantations; and a third group, whose complaints, such as a dislocated shoulder or hernias, were caused by organic disturbances, the witch doctor referred to Dr. Schweitzer. Asked how patients could ever expect to get any good out of a session with a witch doctor, Schweitzer replied, "The witch doctor succeeds for the same reason all the rest of us succeed. Each patient carries his own doctor inside him. They come to us not knowing that truth. We are at our best when we give the doctor who resides within each patient a chance to go to work."

Like Cousins, James Kent, a well-known nineteenth-century homeopathic physician, believed in the value of the placebo. Using homeopathic medicine and a placebo, he cured a case of chronic arthritis in the left knee of a patient. He recognized the success as the value of the body's healing potential and the value of the placebo.

Cousins wrote that the placebo effect was proof that there really was not separation between the mind and the body. In his book *Anatomy of an Illness as Perceived by the Patient: Reflections on Healing and Regeneration*, he recounts many instances of a placebo having a positive effect on healing. He reported that a noted Harvard physician-researcher had found in a review of more than one thousand patients involved in medical studies of illnesses as diverse as headaches, anxiety, and severe postoperative wound pain that 35 percent achieved "satisfactory" relief with a placebo.

Researchers have also studied the placebo effect in patients with arthritis. Cousins reports a study in which 88 patients with arthritis received a placebo rather than standard therapy with cortisone or aspirin. The response of those receiving the placebo was about the same as that of patients receiving conventional therapy. Furthermore, patients who had reported no response with the placebo in pill form

received another round of placebo therapy, this time by injection. Relief
and improvement were reported by 66 percent. All patients reporting
positive results with the placebo said improvement stretched beyond
the arthritis relief, including reductions in swelling, to betterment of
such general aspects of health as sleeping, eating, and bowel habits.

Other physicians have had patients who also used the mind to
escape the pains of the body. Physician Larry Dossey in his book
Meaning and Medicine recounts the story of Walter Dent, a patient in his
nineties whose arthritic knees forced him to rely on a cane in each hand
when he walked. He resolutely refused to take any medication Dossey
prescribed, telling him that he had done just fine for 97 years without
the pills, thank you very much. He charmed the office staff, acting as
confidant and counselor, friend, and cheerful listener. Near his 100th
birthday, the elderly fellow took a spill and broke his hip. Dossey's peer,
an orthopedic specialist called on to perform the surgery, soon was
appealing to Dossey for help in getting the old man to take drugs for
pain relief.

"This guy's got to be in a lot of pain," the surgeon told Dossey," but
I can't get him to take anything for it. Says he has a 'secret' he prefers
to use."

Dent got his way, though, and used his "secret" to escape from the
pain preoperatively and postoperatively. From the outside he seemed to
be sleeping. On the fifth postoperative day, he awoke from his "sleep,"
having never taken any medications for pain relief. When Dossey visited
him, the almost-centenarian was alert and on guard against Dossey's
questions about his intrinsic capability to cope.

"If I told you," he said in response to Dossey's queries about where
he had been, "it wouldn't be a secret, would it?"

Getting More Help

The Arthritis Foundation is probably the best known national
arthritis organization, though other organizations focus on helping
those with such specific disorders as ankylosing spondylitis, lupus,
scleroderma, or Sjögren's syndrome. Visit its Web site *(www.arthritis.
org)*, or call the Arthritis Foundation at 800/283-7800. Correspondence
may be sent to the Arthritis Foundation, P. O. Box 7669, Atlanta, Georgia
30357-0669. The Arthritis Foundation publishes a bimonthly magazine,
Arthritis Today, which reports on arthritis research and treatment and

gives advice to people with arthritis for living a productive pain-free life.

6

When You Need Surgery

"What you should put first...is how to make the patient well; and if he can be made well in many ways, one should choose the least troublesome."—
Hippocrates

*C*an a therapy help you even when you don't know you are practicing it? Consider the case of my patient who underwent arthroscopic knee surgery. When asked about postoperative pain, he told me his wife could relieve the pain he experienced simply by massaging a particular spot on the bottom of his foot. This fellow, who along with his wife had never heard of reflexology, was benefiting from their serendipitous discovery of a formally practiced alternative therapy. Through her desire to support him, she found the nerve ending able to cause the reflex of knee pain relief and to help restore functioning. This type of therapy is related to transcutaneous neural stimulation, in which electrical stimulation of the nerve is used to decrease postoperative pain, which gets patients back on their feet sooner (results of my experiments with this therapy are reported in chapter 7). Avoiding drugs appeals to many patients today, especially women who are pregnant or others who are concerned about drug interactions or side effects. Besides, it feels good.

Fear of knee surgery may not only prevent people from undergoing needed surgery, it may also prevent them from consulting a doctor. When people express anxiety about coming to my office to have their knee evaluated, I tell them, "I promise you, I don't operate in the examining room." Surgery should be the last resort, an option forced on the physician and patient after attempting other solutions. Both need to know that they tried everything reasonable before opting for surgery; nonetheless, a few conditions make surgery inevitable.

Of injuries that are experienced by runners, only about one-fifth of them affect the knees, and most of these are managed without surgical intervention. Many of these injuries can be relieved with changes in activities because, typically, they are the result of overuse from alterations in the pattern of training, equipment, or surface. But many surgical solutions to knee problems are not what are expected. Most people do not realize that about 70 percent of all knee surgery (total knee replacement being the exception) can be performed in less than an hour and on an outpatient basis at an outpatient clinic or the outpatient surgical unit of a hospital.

The most common reason patients visit an orthopedic surgeon is a problem with their knees, according to a 1995—1996 survey by the National Center for Health Statistics. In this survey, knees were a bigger concern than symptoms related to the back, shoulder, hands and fingers, feet and toes, or wrist. In fact, visits for knee symptoms were 1.8 times more common than those for back symptoms, which were the next most common symptom given on the list. Annually, about 624,000 patients in the United States undergo arthroscopy, a minimally invasive surgical procedure to determine what is wrong with their knees. Each year almost 455,000 undergo meniscal surgery, and about 265,000 undergo replacement or other repair of the knee.

For these patients, like all patients undergoing surgery, the process can be stressful. We know that surgery elicits from patients a stress response, triggering a release of hormones responsible in part for a cascade of cardiovascular and metabolic reactions. The heart rate increases, the blood vessels constrict increasing blood pressure, the immune system loses vigor, and organ functions suffer disruption. Anxiety about changes in lifestyle or body image, whether these changes are limited to the postoperative period or expected to stretch beyond it, fuels fears of surgery.

Coping with Surgery

Researchers at the University of California at Davis compare undergoing surgery to running a marathon. They find similarities between the patient's experience and what a runner would feel if told to complete a marathon but given no advice about how to do it—no rules, no standard practices, and no clue of successful strategies. Understandably, they say, "No wonder so many surgical patients feel helpless."

Looking at surgery as something akin to an athletic event offers a useful analogy, and you do not have to be a National Basketball Association star player (or even a fan) to understand it. Like athletic training, preparing for surgery makes you an active participant. You are no longer a passive onlooker. Participation transforms you from someone out of control ("Surgery is something that is done to me") to someone in control ("Surgery is something that is not done without me"). Rehearsal and coaching (self-talk) are also part of this attack on the victim mentality.

For important competitions, athletes are encouraged to rehearse — not only on the court, on the parallel bars, or in the pool, but also in their minds — to imagine the challenges and to imagine how they will meet them. Self-coaching and self-talk, the active dialogue carried on with one's self, can significantly affect outlook. Are you saying to yourself, "I can't believe this is happening to me?" Or are you saying, "I know this will be stressful for me, so I'm going to make a plan for it." Are you saying, "This is too difficult for me?" Or are you saying, "I can do this!"

Even hospitalized children sometimes rehearse procedures or diagnostic tests they may have to undergo. With the help of play therapists, for example, children with cancer may pretend to be part of a bone marrow extraction procedure. They are guided through the steps of the procedure by caring and knowledgeable adults who help them experience in a safe and comfortable playroom environment this part of their treatment. When faced with the real procedure, it is not threateningly foreign or strange. They can say to themselves, "I can do this because I've been through it before."

Presurgical Preparation

Research, not just intuition, tells us that a person's postsurgical recovery is affected by presurgical preparation. Outcome is not simply a result of how serious the ailment is added to the expertise of the surgeon. Many factors are at work, both physical and psychological.

In a study at The University of Texas School of Medicine, my colleagues and I found that nutritional deficiencies can affect outcome significantly. We found that trauma induced a state of malnutrition, and that the depletion found in patients who had suffered trauma or femoral fractures was almost two times that found in patients undergoing hip replacement surgery and 1.6 times that found in patients facing elective surgery. This depletion, which affected patients' ability to prevent infection, was found to relate significantly to the development of complications. Other researchers have also found depressed immune functioning after surgery and linked it to more complicated recoveries. This tells us that we must pay attention to nutrition and its support of the immune system during the crucial recovery and rehabilitation period.

Psychological Preparation

Psychological preparation can also make a difference. It can help the patient meet the challenge of surgery, and the central results of such preparation are reduced postoperative pain and shortened hospitalization. Some of these preparations are conventional (educational information, instructional sessions, and small group therapy) and some are less so (hypnosis or relaxation training). One study at the University of Colorado showed that hospital stays were reduced an average of 2.4 days when patients were psychologically prepared.

Feeling in control when being wheeled into the surgical suite may be difficult to imagine, but planning how to manage your relationships with surgeons and staff, how to work with the options of pain control, and how to manage yourself may be the way to do it.

- **Managing relationships with the surgeon, the anesthesiologist, and staff.** Once you have chosen your surgeon (see suggestions below), you may feel much more comfortable about undergoing the surgery if you prepare a list of questions and get answers to them. You may also have questions for the anesthesiologist.

You will probably want to ask what kind of medication you will be given before you go to the operating room. Not all patients require this preparatory medication, but if you do, the best ones are short acting. The three types of anesthesia used today are safe and should not be rejected out of fear. Local anesthesia prevents the sensation of pain near the incision. Regional anesthesia prevents sensation, for example, throughout the entire leg or below the waist. In these two types, the patient is awake during the procedure. A general anesthesia, in which gas or medications are administered, will make the patient sleep throughout the procedure. Ask about side effects and risks. Ask who will be controlling the anesthesia throughout the surgery. If you have had a negative experience with or a negative reaction to anesthesia, report it to your doctors.

As for the hospital staff, think about what you want from them and make that your aim. If you want efficiency, try to be efficient with them. If you want someone to pat your shoulder or hold your hand for a while, be vocal. Be respectful and usually you'll get respect in return. If you do stay overnight in the hospital, never be reluctant to ask about any new medication you are being asked to take, any tests that are being done, and any limits that may have been set on your activities or diet.

- **Managing pain control.** Be sure to ask your surgeon about medicines to control pain after surgery. Pain control is instrumental following knee surgery to keep the joint moving, which is essential to regaining strength. If you will be hospitalized after the surgery, your hospital may offer patient-controlled anesthesia, which allows you with the push of a thumb to control intravenous (IV) administration of such pain relievers as morphine or meperidine hydrochloride (Demerol) within certain limits. If you are discharged from the hospital or surgery center the same day as your surgery, pain medicine will be prescribed for you to have at home. You can expect an ice cuff or ice bags to be part of the physician's postoperative plan during the first two days after surgery.

- **Managing yourself.** "Know thyself" is a good admonition to keep in mind as you face surgery. What is it about the surgery that worries you? It is better not to deny these fears but to face them and prevent them from hounding you, building up any tension you feel. Remember that you have gains to make from the surgery and that it was good reasoning that brought you to the decision to undergo surgery in the first place. Remind yourself of other difficult situations that you have negotiated, and recapture some of the feelings of success you experienced. Celebrate your ability to make such a serious decision, plan for its consequences, and see it through.

What Your Doctor Can Do

Preparing patients for surgery usually includes giving them educational materials or meeting with them to inform them about what to expect. Surgeons sometimes supply videotapes for patients to view in the office that explain procedures, which may include interviews with patients who have undergone identical or similar procedures. These patients describe their personal response to surgery and how they felt during recovery. Such efforts have been shown by research to sow positive seeds that can be reaped in recovery.

Significant differences have been found between patients who were instructed and patients who were not. Primarily improvements were in reducing the amount of time spent hospitalized and in the amount of pain reported after surgery. Other improvements were in reducing time off from work and circulatory complications.

Less traditional techniques such as hypnosis and relaxation imagery also have been employed to help patients use their minds to relax muscles to control pain and shorten hospitalization. In one study, one of three groups of patients was told that the patients could control muscles in the area near where the incision was made and that it would be profitable to their recovery for them to keep blood away from the area during surgery and to make sure it returned after surgery to nourish the tissues. Their blood loss during surgery was significantly less than that of the other groups.

Participating Intraoperatively

During surgery, when a patient is anesthetized on the table, you may think there is nothing the patient can do; however, some studies are giving patients and surgeons reason to pay attention to what patients hear intraoperatively. Women undergoing hysterectomies who listened to a tape of therapeutic suggestions required less pain medicine postsurgically than did women who listened to a blank tape. In fact, prerecorded tapes made specifically for intraoperative use are commercially available. These tapes mix music with calming reassurances and instructions. But such specially made tapes are not necessary. Whatever music or sounds are relaxing and comforting to the patient should be employed. One study found that the type of music was not as important as patient preference. It could be Bach, rap, heavy metal, or show tunes. When listening to a tape is not a choice you want to make, earplugs may be useful, but the operating team needs to know and approve of your plan to wear them.

Some technical suggestions by Henry Bennett and Elizabeth Disbrow who work at the University of California, Davis, Medical Center, include (1) using a tape player with autoreverse and making sure that feature is turned on; (2) installing fresh batteries; (3) setting the controls and then taping over the buttons to ensure that jolting radio static or broadcasting isn't inadvertently turned on when the patient is moved; and (4) making sure during a prehospitalization visit with the surgeon that using the music and headphones during surgery is preapproved.

Self-hypnosis or self-regulation is another method of dealing with the challenges of surgery. In an interview with journalist Bill Moyers in *Healing and the Mind,* Dr. Karen Olness, a professor of family medicine described how she used self-hypnosis to avoid the pain of a forty-five—minute resuturing of a thumb ligament torn in a skiing accident. Professionally, Dr. Olness teaches children who suffer from migraine headaches how to control the pain by regular practice of a relaxation imagery exercise.

"I must tell you," she told Moyers, "that it was a very reassuring experience, because I had taught this for years, and I wondered whether I could use this technique if I really needed it, and I could." Colleagues videotaped the procedure. She refused anesthesia and shifted her focus and concentration to a familiar and favorite memory of childhood.

"I was extremely comfortable," she said of the experience, "I was perfectly conscious of what was going on outside, but I wasn't very interested in it." Afterward, she compared her accomplishment to winning a competition: "I felt the way I suppose a person does when he or she has finished a marathon. Although it was a mental achievement, my feeling was akin to that of winning a race."

Olness has also worked with children in helping them prepare for surgery. In an experiment, children following specific suggestions to imagine increased immune function were found to have higher levels of immunoglobulins, which are infection-fighting antibodies.

Postoperative Play: Fast-forwarding Recovery

For most patients undergoing knee surgery, controlling pain translates into increased motion, which is essential in fast-forwarding recovery. With regular exercise, the postsurgical knee will increase in strength; without it, recovery may not be complete. From experience, some surgeons have observed a variable "golden" period after surgery during which the body is primed to regain strength. If the patient fails to exercise, strength may plateau at the amount needed for daily routine (about 60%—70%) but not *full* strength.

In a study I performed with colleagues, we used transcutaneous neural stimulation (TNS) and found it to be effective following arthroscopy in reducing postoperative pain and allowing movement of the knee joint. In TNS, the nerves beneath the skin are stimulated. The patients were divided into three groups—a group receiving TNS, a group treated by a "placebo" unit, and a group receiving no treatment. The group undergoing TNS recovered isokinetic power, range of motion, and leg volume in three weeks; it took seven weeks for the other groups to recover to the same level.

But along with obtaining a high level of function, rehabilitation takes into consideration the whole person. Of course, aims for the knee during recuperation should include becoming strong again and certainly avoiding atrophy, improving endurance, and fostering the return of the proprioceptive sense. But other notions of fitness, such as cardiovascular endurance, agility, and unencumbered participation in favorite activities or sports, must also be pursued.

Preparing for surgery is like preparing for an athletic competition. Planning a strategy and mentally rehearsing the hospital admission, the surgery, the postsurgical hospitalization (if any), and discharge will help eliminate many of the worries patients typically carry with them into the operating room. Close your eyes and imagine the best surgical experience and outcome as you define them.

Knee Surgery: What to Expect

It has been more than a generation since a surgical solution to knee problems always meant general anesthesia, a long incision, and an extended recovery period. Below, we examine arthroscopy and three other types of surgical intervention—meniscus repair, knee ligament surgery, and knee replacement.

Arthroscopy

Arthroscopy of the knee is the most commonly performed orthopedic surgical procedure in the United States. Relying on small incisions of less than one-half inch through which instruments and a "scope," or video camera, are inserted, the physician can perform a diagnostic or therapeutic procedure. Therapeutic procedures performed through this minimally invasive surgical method offer patients less swelling, fewer scars, and briefer recovery time than procedures performed with an incision opening the knee to view. Because tests are performed days before the procedure and the anesthetic required is minimal, patients usually do not even stay overnight in the hospital, being admitted and dismissed on the same day. Often the only test required is a complete blood count.

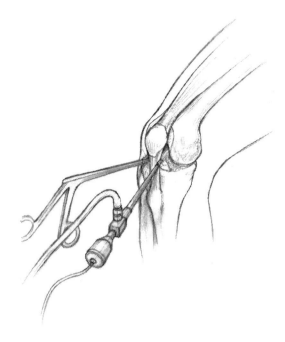

Arthroscopy. With arthroscopy, not only can surgeons inspect the knee's interior, but they can also repair, remove, or reconstruct its parts.

Arthroscopy was originally employed as a way for physicians to determine what was wrong with the knee when an X-ray did not reveal the problem. With the development of new instruments, surgeons were able to add "repair," "remove," and "reconstruct" to the arthroscopy vocabulary of "seeing." Other joints, such as the hip, ankle, and wrist are studied and treated with this technology.

After an orthopedic surgeon evaluates your knee with an examination done in the office or a clinic, he or she may order film studies, including computed axial tomography (CAT) scans or magnetic resonance imaging (MRI) studies, and a preoperative blood test. If the results indicate that your case is appropriate for arthroscopy, you will be scheduled for an outpatient arthroscopy procedure at a hospital or surgical center. MRI studies' improved ability to delineate knee problems has made arthroscopy less essential for diagnosis. Some patients, however, may experience symptoms that are not explained by the MRI, and arthroscopy becomes important in detecting the cause.

Though arthroscopy is minimally invasive, it is still surgery, and you should expect the physician, nurses, and anesthetist to wear masks and be dressed in surgical wear. The anesthesia may be given to the knee area alone (local anesthetic) or to the leg alone (regional anesthetic), numbing the knee but leaving you awake, or it may be given as a general anesthetic, meaning you will sleep throughout the procedure and be awakened after it is over.

After the anesthetic takes effect, your surgeon will make small incisions through which a camera and instruments will be passed. The surgeon will watch a video monitor where what is seen by the camera is projected. The arthroscope uses fiber optic light and magnifying lenses to produce a remarkably clear picture, though training and extensive experience is necessary to be able to navigate with confidence the anatomical topography revealed by the camera. A surgical assistant acts as a camera operator, moving the instrument for better visualization at the surgeon's request while the surgeon, watching the monitor, uses instruments to correct the cause of the knee problem.

The surgeon will be able to diagnose causes of pain, including arthritis, torn ligaments, inflamed tendons, or damaged cartilage. Pieces of bone or cartilage that have broken off and are caught in the joint space (these pieces are called *loose bodies*) can cause popping and clicking as well as pain. Using special instruments, surgeons can repair damaged cartilage or torn ligaments with stitches (sutures) or reattach them or synthetic replacements (still evolving in quality) with screws. They can also remove the loose bodies, a torn meniscus, or synovial membrane overgrowth (common in rheumatoid arthritis). Sports injuries may require reconstruction of ligaments (see below).

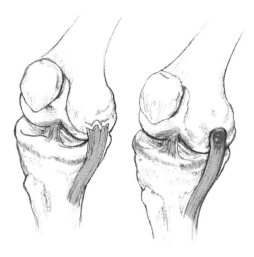

Ligament repair. Surgeons sometimes reattach torn ligaments with screws.

Meniscus Repair

Injury to the half-moon—shaped cartilage called the *meniscus* that acts as a shock absorber within the knee is the most frequent cause for knee arthroscopic surgery. Injury during activity often results in a meniscus tear in a young person, and some physicians have suggested increasingly demanding sports as a reason. In older people, osteoarthritis and the more vulnerable condition of the meniscus make it prone to injury. According to government statistics, patients who have to undergo this surgery are most likely to be between 15 and 44 years old.

Pain, knee instability, and fluid on the knee are consequences of meniscal injuries. Using arthroscopy, the surgeon can assess the injury and remove loose pieces of meniscal cartilage. Long-term studies have indicated that patients in whom the meniscus could be preserved were at lower risk of disability from early degenerative changes.

Recognizing the importance of the meniscus to knee health and stability, surgeons and scientists are working to support meniscus preservation, healing, and—in experimental studies—regeneration. New technology, expanding life expectancies, and more active middle age and elder lifestyles are driving these efforts. Surgeons exercise surgical restraint, repair ruptures or tears with suturing, and even transplant menisci harvested from donors. Brown University scientists showed in a preliminary study that a collagenous biomaterial derived from pigs could be deposited in a meniscal tear in a rabbit and promote regeneration.

Knee Ligament Surgery

Of the four ligaments bracing your knee, two are more likely than the others to be injured: the anterior cruciate ligament and the medial collateral ligament. The anterior cruciate ligament, connecting thighbone (femur) to shinbone (tibia) in the center of the knee, is prone to be injured when the knee is twisted dramatically, as sometimes happens during skiing. When the anterior cruciate ligament is torn, the injured person can sense more play in the knee than formerly. Other injury often accompanies an anterior cruciate ligament injury. The medial collateral ligament, connecting femur to tibia on the side of the inner knee, is supposed to limit the sideways movement of the knee and is injured most often by impact. A force hits the outside of the knee, forcing the medial collateral ligament governing the inside of the knee to be stretched beyond normal bounds. The injury may escalate beyond a stretch to a partial or complete tear. You may hear a pop, and your knee may give way.

Both of these injuries impair your mobility, and both, if left untreated, can open the door to greater problems. Get help promptly if you suspect you have one of these injuries. Pain and swelling should be treated with an ice pack, which should help reduce both. Your level of physical activity and the degree of injury will affect your physician's decision about whether to treat your problem surgically or nonsurgically. Factors in the decision include determining whether any other tissue is injured, evaluating the demands your lifestyle places on your knee, and estimating the possibility of re-injury.

If the physician decides surgical treatment is best, your anterior cruciate ligament will be reconstructed with a graft (replacement tissue) from a tendon in the knee, with synthetic material, or with an allograft (tendon from a cadaver). Allografts are sometimes rejected by the body and have in some cases been linked with synovitis, an infection; however, patients benefit by not having to donate the tissue themselves. Your surgeon will use arthroscopy to determine the extent of the injury and to find any additional injuries. When the patient and surgeon decide to use a graft from the patient, the surgeon will obtain the graft through a small incision after drilling holes in the tibia and femur where the graft will be attached. The graft is threaded through the holes and attached at each end with screws. The surgeon may add another tendon to supplement support.

If your physician decides surgical treatment is best for your medial collateral ligament, the procedure will begin with an arthroscopic examination to determine if there are additional injuries within the joint. Often, injuries to the anterior cruciate ligament or the meniscus accompany an injury to the medial collateral ligament. Although these torn parts can be repaired arthroscopically, the medial collateral ligament repair, which involves screwing, stapling, or stitching your ligament back together, must be performed with traditional open surgery involving a long incision. When there are no other injuries, physicians usually opt for nonsurgical treatment of a medial collateral ligament, allowing the ligament to heal by itself. This approach requires controlling the swelling, resting the joint by not putting any weight on it, and exercising it through a planned graduated program intended at first to promote healing and later to reestablish range of motion and to rebuild strength and flexibility.

Both types of surgeries require general anesthesia and a two- or three-day postoperative hospitalization. The risks and complications inherent in surgical procedures accompany both. A commitment to rehabilitation through a planned program of physical therapy and home exercises is necessary to achieve the best possible results from either procedure. During the immediate postoperative recovery period, the focus will be on enhancing the healing process by reducing pain and swelling and using a continuous passive motion (CPM) machine for exercise. A CPM machine helps promote drainage of your knee, which reduces swelling and pain, and moves your joint gently, keeping it from getting stiff and propelling you forward in your rebuilding exercise program. The CPM machine can be used in the hospital, in the physical therapist's office, or at home.

Total Knee Replacement

Total knee replacement may be necessary when arthritis, an injury, poor alignment, or just plain old wear and tear cause knee pain and stiffness that interfere with or prevent you from participating in normal activities. Simple walking can be very painful, and a flight of stairs can loom as an impossibility. Arthritic conditions for which total knee replacement is appropriate include osteoarthritis, which can break down the joint cartilage that cushions your knee, and rheumatoid arthritis, in which inflammation and swelling make joints painful to move. Total knee replacement involves resurfacing the bones of the knee joint to improve joint movement. It can involve from one to three joint surfaces within the knee. In some cases, unicompartmental knee surgery, which is limited to replacing a part rather than the whole knee, is an option.

In total knee replacement, an artificial knee joint, called a *prosthesis,* is custom tailored to your needs. The prosthesis will replace one, two, or three surfaces of the knee joint. Because total knee replacement carries the risks and possibility of complications of any complex orthopedic procedure, your physician will recommend replacement only after carefully examining you and evaluating your X-rays and any other studies ordered. Total knee replacement seems to benefit mostly those who are older than 60 years of age, who weigh less than 250 pounds, who do not have vascular disease in their legs, and who have pain that prevents them from participating in normal daily activities. Having a total knee replacement will not restore knee function completely; some restrictions will apply, but the pain relief it provides will permit return to some activities that had to be given up because of problems with the knee. Knee prostheses cannot hold up under participation in some sports and some heavy work, and the normal life span of a prosthesis is only 10 to 15 years.

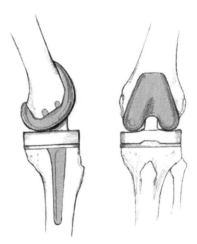

Total knee replacement. In total knee replacement, surgeons resurface the bones of the knee joint to improve joint movement. In some cases, surgery can be limited to replacing a part rather than the whole knee. The prosthesis, or artificial knee joint, has smooth surfaces similar to those of a normal knee.

Presurgical tests for all patients will include a complete blood count, a blood chemistry study, a magnetic resonance imaging study, and a bone scan, and for patients who are more than forty years old, a chest X-ray and electrocardiogram will be added. Only rarely is an arthrogram necessary. An arthrogram is an X-ray study that uses dye called opaque contrast material within the joint to help identify tears.

Total knee replacement takes two to three hours and begins with an incision that is initiated above the knee and ends about four to six inches below the kneecap. The surgeon will shape the bone surfaces to ensure the best fit with the prosthesis. The three components of a total knee replacement are the femoral component that caps the end of your thighbone, the tibial component that resurfaces the top of the shin bones, and the patellar component that fits underneath the kneecap.

After surgery, the knee will be covered with a large bandage and a drain will be in place to provide an outlet for postoperative bleeding. The health care team at the hospital will engage you in easy exercises initially and then move you forward to the physical therapy necessary to gain as much use as possible from your new knee. Over time, you will progress from walking with a walker to walking with crutches and then to walking with a cane. Even at home, physical therapy may remain part of a planned recovery program that integrates home exercises with professional care.

What's Up, Doc? Questions to Ask Your Surgeon

All patients have questions about any surgical procedure they have been asked to undergo. Writing down these questions and taking them with you to the doctor's office can help ensure that you don't come home afterward and discover that in the haste of the examination you forgot to ask the questions most important to you. When you choose your surgeon, you may want recommendations not only from patients but also from other physicians. Even if you are part of a managed care program, you will probably have a choice of providers. In addition to the questions on your list, consider asking those below:

- How successful is the procedure you are recommending?
- Will the benefits outweigh the risks?
- Are you comfortable performing this procedure?
- What procedures do you perform most often?
- Do you specialize in a specific type of surgery?
- What kind of complications should I expect?

- What can I expect from my knee after the surgery?
- What has been the outcome in other patients in your practice who have undergone this surgery?

Surgery Scenarios

Patients may have an immediate reaction to the suggestion of surgery. Here are a few scenarios coupled with a professional response.

"The doctor said I need surgery, but I don't. My mother's cousin had this same problem, and she never even went to a doctor."

Determining whether you need surgery or not by similar ailments suffered by family members fails to take into account the unique nature of your knees. Going to another physician is a better tactic. The first doctor you consult may be willing to recommend a second. Some insurance companies even pay part of the cost of obtaining a second opinion. Do be wary if when obtaining a second opinion, a surgeon urges immediate action. Make sure you understand why—that the surgeon can specify the consequences of postponing the surgery—and call the physician you first consulted to find out if he or she shares this concern. Of course, you can always ask, "What will happen if I don't have this surgery?"

"I am not going to have this done in a community hospital or an outpatient center. I want the best care and that means going to the medical center."

It is true that in large medical centers there are concentrations of well-trained physicians and well-equipped hospitals offering excellent surgical support; however, consider whether the procedure you'll be undergoing is complicated or not. Teaching hospitals, centers where medical school students and graduates are working, are considered excellent, as are some public hospitals where some of the best and the brightest of medical students go for broad experience. Are there potential risks related to the complexity of the procedure, or are there unknowns about your case that would require the expertise found in a medical center? If you conclude that your knee surgery is straightforward and determine that your surgeon is board certified and handles this type of case routinely, the community hospital may offer competent patient care at a lower cost.

All patients should consider outpatient ambulatory surgery centers. Today, outpatient centers are an excellent option for patients requiring all types of surgery, from complicated, time-consuming joint replacements to routine, straight-forward arthroscopies. Many patients find that having surgery at an outpatient center costs less, is more accommodating, and is more comfortable. Research also shows that outpatient centers have lower infection rates than hospitals, thus improving your chances of a quick recovery. Ask your physician about having your procedure done in an outpatient center, and research the facility he recommends — the best ones are certified by the Accreditation Association for Ambulatory Health Care, or "AAAHC Certified." Visit *www.aaahc.org* to search for accredited facilities.

Foremost, be comfortable with your surgeon, and make choosing your surgeon your first priority. Knee surgery is not considered risky unless the patient has other conditions that complicate care; therefore, it is commonly performed in community and suburban hospitals.

"Those diagnostic tests are unending — twenty-four hours a day. That's all they do is stick you."

With some knee procedures, you will not stay overnight in the hospital, so there is no reason to worry about the threat of feeling like a pincushion. For simple arthroscopy, a complete blood count (CBC) may be the only test required. A total knee replacement, though, will require a CBC and more: possibly a urinalysis, a chest X-ray, and an electrocardiogram, depending on age and coexisting conditions. Blood chemistry, an MRI, and a bone scan will probably be requested. In rare cases, surgeons want an arthrogram (an X-ray study made of your knee after dye has been injected in the joint).

Depending on how the hospital is organized, you may be able to have all your preoperative evaluations performed in one area in the hospital devoted to preoperative testing. Other hospitals may perform all the tests under their roof, but you may have to move from unit to unit to have tests done.

"I am not having a blood transfusion. No way."

Blood supply experts tell us that the blood supply is extremely safe. In most knee procedures, blood is rarely needed because of the use of a tourniquet placed above the knee. Blood transfusion is usually only needed in cases of total knee replacement. Discuss your concerns with your doctor. One option some patients chose is donating their own blood before the surgery. This is called an *autologous* blood donation. The hospital stores it and has it on hand in case a transfusion is needed. If it is not needed, the blood may be used like any other donation.

Another option is the cell saver machine used in operating rooms to recycle the blood a patient loses during surgery.

7

Mind-Body Connections and Knee Health: Alternative, or Complementary, Medicine

"The natural healing force within each one of us is the greatest force in getting well." —Hippocrates

*S*ometimes pain unrelated to a physical ailment can become focused in a joint. Not too long ago, a Southwestern Native American leader came to see me because of pain in his left shoulder. He complained of gradually increasing pain and stiffness in his shoulder that had eventually resulted in experiencing pain with even the smallest movement of his shoulder. Doctors call this frozen shoulder. A condition in the knee that is similarly painful and limiting is arthrofibrosis.

Because coronary artery disease produces angina that feels like it is radiating into the left shoulder and arm and because this patient's age and sex alone put him at risk of heart disease, I began asking him questions about any problems he might have experienced previously with his heart. He told a story of formerly being hospitalized near his home for heart surgery. Hours before the surgery, shamans from his tribe assembled in his room and through a native ceremony determined that his heart pain was at least in part due to his lingering grief over the loss of his wife, who had died a short time before. The religious leaders addressed this grief in their ceremony.

After their intercession, the leader was relieved of his pain, and he left the hospital without undergoing surgery. After hearing this account and determining through my own evaluation that the leader's current shoulder problem was not caused by coronary artery disease, I assured him that a therapist could help him learn to exercise the shoulder to gradually relieve the tension and pain. In addition, I encouraged him to seek the wisdom of his tribe's shamans again, believing that his unresolved grief over his wife's death—heart pain of a different sort—could be part of the discomfort he was experiencing.

Public and professional attitudes toward alternative and complementary medicine have undergone remarkable changes in the last 10 years. Not only are more patients turning to alternative and complementary therapies, but also many report that they now feel more comfortable in discussing unconventional treatments with their doctors. According to a survey published in the *Journal of the American Medical Association* in November 1998, the number of Americans who have used alternative or complementary therapies rose from 33 percent in 1990 to 42 percent in 1997. That same year, Americans spent more than $27 billion on herbal medicines, massage, megavitamins, and other unconventional therapies—an amount greater than what was spent that year on out-of-pocket hospital expenses.

Reasons for this change in tide rest in consumers' aversion to the high technology, high cost, and low personalization of American medicine. Such unconventional therapies as massage, biofeedback, and relaxation techniques are more understandable and more accessible than CAT and MRI scans, and practitioners of alternative medicine, in comparison to conventional providers, spend more time with patients—in fact, one study found that they spend about twice as much time.

But just because those patients using unconventional medicine are resisting high-tech, high-cost health care doesn't mean they are uneducated. One study found that people who seek alternative health care providers typically are 25 to 49 years old, and while all socioeconomic groups are represented among users, most have relatively more education and higher incomes than the general population.

The Uneasy Truce: A "Don't Ask, Don't Tell" Policy

Physicians, understandably, have been slower to accept or even acknowledge alternative and complementary therapies. After all, until very recently, well-conducted clinical trials of unconventional therapies were virtually nonexistent. In the absence of this rigid scientific scrutiny—and with little or no exposure to alternative medicine in medical school—many traditional physicians have been reluctant to endorse unconventional techniques. The result has been an uneasy "don't ask, don't tell" policy, whereby patients who use these treatments have not asked about them and have not divulged their practice, using them on the sly.

But that, too, appears to be changing. *Consumer Reports* magazine in May 2000 published results of a survey of more than 46,000 of its readers that asked about their use of alternative and complementary medicine. A surprising finding was that nearly one quarter of the survey respondents said they had tried an unconventional treatment on the recommendation of a doctor or a nurse. About 60 percent of the respondents who had turned to alternatives reported that they had shared that information with their doctors. (In the 1998 *Journal of the American Medical Association* survey, respondents reported that they did *not* discuss about 60 percent of their unconventional treatments with their doctors.) In the *Consumer Reports* survey, 55 percent of respondents said their doctors had responded favorably to the shared information, 40 percent reported a neutral response, and only 5 percent said their doctors had expressed disapproval.

Several factors have contributed to these changing attitudes. The establishment of the Office of Alternative Medicine (OAM) at the National Institutes of Health (NIH) in 1992 was a landmark, but it was a very controversial event. Originally a small entity within the NIH Office of the Director, the OAM has evolved into a full-fledged center at NIH—the National Center for Complementary and Alternative Medicine (NCCAM). From a near-token annual budget of $2 million in fiscal year 1993, the NCCAM budget had grown to $68.7 million by 2000. The NCCAM, which divides alternative and complementary medicine into five domains (see chart), funds research that will answer questions about effectiveness.

Conventional Medicine's Journals and Unconventional Medicine's Research

The NCCAM expansion has given greater leeway to its research endeavors, giving the American people something they haven't had until now—a reliable source of information about a confusing and, for the most part, unregulated area of medical treatment. Some critics of alternative medicine believe the NIH affiliation gives these therapies a degree of respect that has not been earned. Others welcome the opportunity for alternative treatments to be put to the test in stringent clinical trials.

This is, in fact, happening. Increasingly, well-respected medical journals are reporting studies of complementary and alternative therapies. As is true with conventional medical treatments, some therapies appear to have merit, whereas others have proved to be of little value. One of the first well-conducted American trials of an herbal medicine was published in *JAMA,* the *Journal of the American Medical*

Association, in 1997. In that study, people with mild dementia who took ginkgo biloba showed modest improvements on tests of cognitive skills. In a study of St. John's wort, reported in the *British Medical Journal* about three years later, the herb was found to be as effective as the conventional prescription medication imipramine in relieving mild to moderate depression—and it had fewer side effects. Similarly, when researchers reporting in the *Journal of the American Medical Association* in March 2000 analyzed several studies of glucosamine and chondroitin for osteoarthritis, they found some evidence of benefit. New studies and additional analyses of existing studies will further contribute to our understanding of its effects and its limitations.

As expected, along with these positive results have come reports suggesting potential dangers. St. John's wort, for example, has been shown to interfere with the metabolism of several types of prescription medications, and researchers found evidence that ginkgo biloba can increase bleeding in patients taking blood-thinners—problems that underscore the importance of open and honest doctor-patient communication concerning alternative remedies. Some physicians have expressed concern about cancer patients' use of large doses of vitamin C and other antioxidants, which can blunt the cell-killing effects of radiation therapy and chemotherapy. Similar worries surround the popular use of soy isoflavone supplements to prevent breast cancer. Some evidence suggests that high doses of these plant-based estrogens can have the opposite effect, potentially fueling the growth of existing, but undiagnosed, breast cancers. Safety, with good reason, remains a primary concern of many physicians who are reluctant to embrace unproven therapies and remains the best reason to discuss all alternative medicine use with your doctor.

Nonetheless, some—and perhaps many—complementary therapies will prove to be valuable additions to conventional medical treatments. Some therapies—such as acupuncture, acupressure, biofeedback, and meditation—are already accepted treatments for certain medical problems. Tomorrow's physicians undoubtedly will be more knowledgeable about unconventional therapies. Once nonexistent, medical school courses on complementary medicine are common today. In fact, a study published in 1998 found that 75 of the nation's 117 medical schools offered elective courses in the subject or included the topic in required courses. Moreover, many of the nation's most respected medical institutions now have complementary medicine departments or centers.

Meeting the Challenge of Choice

For now, the challenge for patients and physicians alike is to remain both open-minded and cautious when using or recommending alternative and complementary therapies. Well-conducted, peer-reviewed research into each technique's potential benefits and risks is critical. Quality control issues, especially questions concerning the purity and standardization of herbs and other supplements, remain a concern and ultimately may necessitate government oversight. For example, the NCCAM cites on its Web site (*http://nccam.nih.gov/*) a *Los Angeles Times* story that reported finding that the potency of 10 St. John's wort products varied dramatically from that reported on their labels and recommended that consumers buy products labeled "standardized extract."

While we wait for the dust of ongoing studies to settle, I consider all treatment options—whether traditional or alternative—as *complementary*, and I follow a whole-person model of healing. When we think about how we treat minor ailments within our families, we find that same whole-person model. No parent attending to a child's scraped knee would fail to ask how the child felt, not offer "to kiss and make it better," and give the child a pat on the back or a hug. In treating a knee condition, a surgeon would be remiss to think that only surgically repairing a cartilage tear or other injury fully rehabilitates the patient. Attention must always be given to the complete person—mind, body, and spirit.

Children still sing the song about the knee bone being connected to the thighbone and the thighbone being connected to the hipbone and so on. Educators tell us that when young children first draw pictures, they do not hesitate to put the sun and the moon in the same sky in one picture. Their world is a whole world, not one with discrete parts acting independently. What children accept instinctively and what the interest in these complementary therapies says is that, though we may not clearly understand how, the mind and the body do interact and emotions, outlook, our sense of self, and our physical being are intertwined.

Consequently, in my practice, I prefer to think of all treatment options, whether traditional or alternative, as not mutually exclusive—not strictly *alternative* treatments but *complementary* ones. At times, the classic Western treatment can be merged with alternative therapy. That people from around the world travel to the United States for medical treatment is an index to the exceptional care available here, and merging that care with successful alternative therapies can offer the best of all worlds.

Many alternative therapies were originally conceived as preventive measures, and "treatments" don't even have to be treatments per se. "Life itself is bigger than illness, diagnosis, treatment or disease mechanism," according to physician Matthew Budd. "A moment of laughter, a walk in the country, simple touching, or tears can reorganize biology in a way that drugs cannot." Below I describe some complementary therapies to provide at least a brief introduction so that those that appeal may be investigated further.

Avoiding the Either-Or Mindset

Evaluating an alternative therapy as a complement to traditional treatment is an option any patient can exercise. But it takes work. The message here is not "Be an alternative medicine enthusiast or be square." The message is "Take responsibility for your health." That means making sure that you have a diagnosis that makes sense to you, a treatment that corrects the problem and brings relief of symptoms and pain, and a plan for continued relief, rehabilitation, or both. Don't neglect the fabulous benefits of Western medicine, but do not reject a complementary therapy that is safe and meets a need just because it isn't mainstream. Working with both types of medicine offers the best of both worlds.

The ABC's of Alternative and Complementary Medicine

Below are some ABC's of alternative and complementary medicine, which include descriptions of how these therapies have been used to remedy knee problems.

Acupuncture

Acupuncture is hardly new. It has been practiced in China for over two thousand years with success. Its aim is to restore the balance of vital energy and to sustain or reestablish normal mind-body functioning. Acupuncturists insert tiny thin needles approximately 12 to 37 centimeters in length under the skin at specific meridian points and at specific depths to accomplish such goals as relieving pain or curing disease. Acupuncture can be used to block both acute and chronic pain, whether from a surgical procedure or muscle spasm. Over twenty states license acupuncturists, and some insurance companies are beginning to cover their treatments. A leader in the state of Washington voted to require insurance companies to cover acupuncture treatments beginning in 1996. Acupuncturists use needles to stimulate various pressure points and restore the flow of *chi* energy along the meridians relevant to the problem. The Chinese define *chi* as the vital life force pervading all things. Health depends on whether *chi* flows freely through the body. This can be done by warming the needle heads, by twirling the needles, or by adding a low electrical pulse to them. Incorporating the herb moxa into the acupuncture process to supplement the energy is called *moxibustion*. The Western explanation for how acupuncture works (as opposed to the eastern theory of *chi*) is that the needles stimulate potent analgesic-packing proteins (endorphins) and opiate- and analgesic-linked pentapeptides (enkephalins) found in the brain.

Two case reports serve as examples of patients with knee problems who found help in acupuncture. The first was a 55-year-old man with moderate arthritis in his knee. He also had a stomach condition that prevented his taking anti-inflammatory medicine. He could exercise some but not much because of knee pain. X-ray films of his knee showed some arthritis, but that alone and his symptoms were not serious enough to require total knee replacement. His case was in that gray area—his problems demanded more than a do-nothing-and-wait approach but his problems were not serious enough to make him a surgical candidate. Acupuncture filled the bill. It has sustained him for about five years. An advantage of postponing total knee replacement is that a patient can get better while waiting. I tell many people that this is staged therapy and that it will help for a certain amount of time and quite possibly forever.

Another patient was a 30-year-old woman who had undergone knee surgery. A skin nerve was cut as it commonly is, but for some reason she developed a neuroma—a chronic inflammation of the nerve. Massage, injections, and other interventions did not improve her condition. She averted surgical re-exploration of the knee by opting for acupuncture, which was successful in curing the problem.

If you see an acupuncturist, be sure he or she is qualified. Licensing varies and, in fact, some physicians trained in U.S. medical schools are also acupuncturists. You should always be sure that the acupuncturist uses presterilized needles. Contact the following organizations for more information: the American Association of Oriental Medicine (*http://www.aaom.org*) (433 Front Street, Catasauqua, Pennsylvania 18032-2506; 610/266-1433), the National Commission for the Certification of Acupuncture and Oriental Medicine (*http://www.nccaom.org*) (11 Canal

Center Plaza, Suite 300; Alexandria, Virginia 22314; 703/548-9004), and the Accreditation Commission for Acupuncture and Oriental Medicine *(http://www.acaom.org)* (7501 Greenway Center Drive, Suite 820; Greenbelt, Maryland 20770; 301/313-0855). The American Academy of Medical Acupuncture, founded in 1987, is the only acupuncture organization in North America that requires its members to be physicians, although it accepts members from a range of training settings. Its Web site may be found at *http://www.medicalacupuncture. org.*

Acupressure (Shiatsu)

Similar to acupuncture but practiced much longer, acupressure uses the hands or feet to gently put pressure on the same points as prescribed in acupuncture. (There are about 125 acupressure points.) Conceived as a way to help the body heal itself, acupressure was initiated approximately five thousand years ago by the Chinese. A few tips about evaluating acupressure: Only gentle pressure should be used. It should not cause lingering pain. Some points would be forbidden during pregnancy. Never undergo acupressure under the influence of alcohol or soon after eating, and sit or lie down after treatment.

Acupressure is a broader term that encompasses some other types of hand massage therapy. *Shiatsu* literally means "finger pressure." This is massage—a rhythmic pushing, stretching, and tapping—for a few seconds at different acupuncture meridian points. Jin Shin uses acupuncture points at specific meridian points and channels. The pressure is held for one to five minutes. Forms of this are called Jin Shin Jyutso, Jin Shin Jitsu, and Jin Shin Do. Another type is Tui Na. This again is a Chinese massage but with a wider variation of hand movements at the pressure points.

Acupressurists are not specially licensed; however, many licensed massage therapists know how to do these types of treatments.

Autogenic Training

Autogenic training combines assuming a relaxed state with mind-body awareness meant to promote self-fulfillment and to extend or expand abilities. In pain control, it is a technique meant to eliminate pain by refocusing concentration. For example, if you are having a lot of pain in your right knee, focus your complete attention on your left knee. Touch your pain-free knee. Move your knee. Feel the normal sensation of movement that is without pain. Feel the normal amount of warmth or coolness that it has. Feel the weight of your leg. Does it feel light or does it feel heavy? Then start focusing on your breathing and your heart rate, trying to allow these to become slow and regular. This exercise will help you redirect your concentration from the painful knee to the rest of your body.

Ayurvedic Medicine

Ayurvedic medicine, the traditional medicine of India, has been practiced for over six thousand years and its name means "the science of life." The universal life energy is called *prana*. Similar to other systems that seek a balance of energy within and without, it is expressed in bipolar terms, Shiva-Shakti, which is equivalent to yin and yang in traditional Chinese medicine. In this discipline, therapies, medicines, and diseases are all classified in this plus-and-minus, warm-and-cold, strong-weak system. *Tridosha* is a fundamental principle that divides healing into humors. These are air *(vata),* fire *(pitta),* water *(kapha),* and ether. Excessive physical strain or injury can intensify the air humor. Within the injury can be inflammation, or part of the fire humor. One treatment for the derangement of the air humor is Narayana oil, which is named after the Hindu god Vishnu. This oil has been used in India for painful joints.

Biofeedback

Biofeedback in its simplest form is the body check referred to in chapter 2. In other words, it is sensing your body and manipulating some involuntary process (heart rate, muscle tension, or temperature, for example) by conscious effort. Modern technology has aided this age-old practice by easily showing biofeedback's effect through graphic displays and digital read-outs. Unquestionably, it is easier to appreciate the ability to auto regulate our bodies by seeing it on a video monitor or hearing it. I was amazed to find that with a $10 biofeedback temperature sensor I could instantly measure a change of temperature in my finger induced by biofeedback technique.

Essentially any bodily function that we can measure is applicable to biofeedback techniques — the brain waves of an electroencephalograph, heart rate on a monitor, or temperature indicated on a thermometer, for instance. The more complex the problem, the more training in relaxation and biofeedback techniques required. The Biofeedback Certification Institute can help identify and locate a certified practitioner.

One indication that conventional medicine is beginning to recognize biofeedback's virtues came in 1996. In a report in the

Journal of the American Medical Association, the National Institutes of Health Technology Assessment Panel on Integration of Behavioral and Relaxation Approaches into the Treatment of Chronic Pain and Insomnia recognized biofeedback's role in relieving chronic pain. Though it said the technique's effect on improving the ability to fall asleep and improving total sleep time may not have been statistically significant, biofeedback was cited for providing improvements in some aspects of sleep.

I've sent more than one patient for biofeedback treatment, only to find out in the counseling component that there was a significant underlying emotional problem adding to the pain. This emphasizes once again how all these treatment options must be blended together, and discussing emotional distress may be important to finding the right treatment.

Botanical Medicine

Botanical medicine is the science and art of using plants to prevent, alleviate, or cure disease. Any plant with healing properties is called an herb. Herbal medicine is essentially as old as mankind. Linoleic, linolenic, and arachidonic acids—three fatty acids essential to human nutrition—are found in plants. There are three-quarters of a million known plants in the world, of which we know also a small quantity have herbal qualities. With greater study of herbs in the rain forest, even more will become available. Of course, these are used in traditional medicine as well. From digitalis, or foxglove, come the cardiac stimulant digitalis and the cardiotonic steroid digoxin. In South America, efforts to make it more profitable for the natives to leave the rain forest for potential drug development rather than clear cutting it appear to be making headway.

One "healer" in San Miguel, Mexico, gave me a tip for using aloe vera. She combined the healing properties of aloe vera with ice and massage by buying aloe vera emollient in liquid or gel, freezing it, and applying it with massage. You can freeze it in a paper cup, tear part of the paper away, and (holding it with the bottom of the cup still in place) use it as an ice massage on the irritated area. I subsequently used this on patients with good results. A plant with analgesic effects, white willow bark, can be used like aspirin because its active ingredient—salicylic acid—is the same.

Breathing Therapy

You can hardly get any argument today against the proposition that breathing is good. An extension of normal inhalation, deep breathing is a conscious effort to completely expand the lungs and relax while giving a super oxygen "fix" to the body. Concentrated breathing practice may last for as few as five minutes a day and is often used as a prelude or postlude to other exercise.

In various disciplines, such as transcendental meditation and yoga, rhythmic deep breathing with controlled inhalation and exhalation is practiced to relieve stress, improve focus, and achieve a somewhat altered state of consciousness. Like hyperventilation, slow deep breathing can evoke changes in brain wave activity that can be monitored by electroencephalography. On a simpler level, aimed at achieving relaxation, patients can pair exercises (slowly rolling the head right or left, rolling the shoulders forward or backward, swinging arms forward or backward) with inhaling (movement one way) and exhaling (movement the other). Pursing the lips to exhale instead of exhaling through the nose slows the exhalation rate and helps ensure complete emptying of the lungs.

Chi

I was fortunate to be team physician for the first football game in China played at Shenzhen. On this fascinating trip I learned first-hand about Oriental medicine and specifically the understanding of *chi*. Because *chi* is very abstract, it is difficult to define. I am reminded of the Native American understanding of the "Great Spirit." This Great Spirit permeates all things from rocks, to people, to energy. *Chi* is essentially the consolidation and expansion of energy, the balance of internal and external forces, the universal energy that exists in all things. It has been discussed as the lifeline or force that makes up one's mind and body.

The Chinese believe that *chi* flows throughout the human body. Health reflects an easy, balanced flow of *chi*. If there is some blockage of *chi* by a body part or organ, health disruption, disease, illness, fatigue, and/or stress can ensure. Taoists believe the universe was originally a ball of *chi*. Around this *chi* was essentially entropy, or random order— the opposite of condensation of *chi*—or chaos. When all of this energy settled out, it divided into yin and yang, the yin (female) being the negative or dark or interior energy and the yang (male) being the positive or light or exterior energy. When one is healthy and the *chi* is flowing easily, the yin and yang are balanced. *Chi* flows through the body through fourteen different meridians. These meridians along with organs are the Eastern corollaries to Western anatomy and physiology.

A knee injury and its resultant pain may block the flow of *chi* through the body. Even if this injury results in a permanent physical disability, the aim is to restore the flow of *chi* through the knee. If in an effort to get in shape, a patient becomes exercise compulsive and fails to pay attention to pain in the knee, tendonitis may result. In therapy, the aim would be to first put the life back in balance (control the compulsivity) and then the flow of *chi* would be restored and the tendonitis would resolve.

Chiropractic Medicine

The word *chiropractic* means "treating with the hands." When looking for a doctor of chiropractic medicine, you should determine if he or she is licensed. Many chiropractors have individual techniques of manipulation and adjustment. The original nineteenth-century therapy by grocer David D. Palmer was that when the spine was subtly out of alignment, it could be adjusted and the conditions resulting from the misalignment resolved. Occasionally nerve or disk dysfunction in the back is the cause of knee pain; therefore, treating the back can alleviate knee pain. However, adjustments for subluxations of the patella or the knee will not work because these are often due to a muscle-ligament imbalance and can only be corrected by muscle strengthening and/or surgical reconstruction of the ligaments. I have seen a few patients who have had well-intended but ineffective "readjustments" of a knee because it "kept going out of place." In fact, this was not the type of subtle subluxation or ligament creep seen in the spine or some other joints; rather, it was the loss of integrity of a ligament, such as the anterior cruciate ligament, in the knee.

Hydrotherapy

It shouldn't be any wonder that a body composed of two-thirds water could be benefited by water in healing. The early Greek physicians knew this, as did James Currie, in 1797, who wrote about the effects of water, cold and warm. The use of water in various forms, baths with additives, for example, has been championed by many people with great success. When we talk about hydrotherapy, we are really talking about the additives in the water, the pulsation of the water, and the temperature of the water.

If you abruptly injure your knee, you need to apply ice or ice water to your knee. This reduces the blood flow to the area, which in turn will decrease the amount of potential inflammation. The coolness also serves as an anesthetic to decrease pain. However, if the ice is left on for too long (greater than 20 minutes at a time), a reflex basal dilatation, or opening up of the blood vessels, may occur. The body part thinks it is freezing and therefore tries to put more blood flow in this area; therefore, this can have a reverse effect and cause more swelling. I like the use of ice bags as opposed to synthetic ice packs because synthetic packs (especially when strapped to the area with an Ace bandage) can actually result in a burn at the numbed area.

Warm water can be used to stimulate circulation and healing. Unfortunately, as mentioned above, warmth can also bring some inflammation, especially if the area is already inflamed. Many different compounds can be added to the warm water to aid in relaxation of the body part and also possibly increase perspiration. Epsom salts tend to relax the area and increase perspiration. A whirlpool combines heat and pressure, producing the positive benefits of a "water massage." But those with an injured knee or other part should take care not to expose it too closely to the pulsation because more bruising could result.

I like to use ice water or ice initially on the injury until the swelling stabilizes, sometime between 24 to 72 hours. After stabilization occurs, I use what trainers recommend, and that is contrast therapy. This is five minutes of heat followed by five minutes of ice followed by five minutes of heat and then five minutes of ice. This is repeated later in the day. This alternating therapy combines the effects of the ice with the healing of heat but stops the inflammation from returning by repeating the ice.

Hypnosis

When you think of hypnosis, you may think of a parlor trick in which someone does something and later has no recollection of it. This is actually far from the case with hypnosis. Usually someone hypnotized can break out of the hypnotic state at any point. The American Society of Clinical Hypnosis reports that there are 15,000 people practicing this technique. Behavioral modification therapists use it to change many different types of behavior.

Experts are not sure how it works. It may manipulate the limbic system, that part of the brain controlling emotion and motivation, allowing the subject to be open to suggestion. Hypnosis can be used for pain (such as that caused by arthritis) by essentially disassociating the mind from the body's pain. Some theories of how arthritis pain can be taken away evolve around the perception that the patient can get amnesia and therefore forget periods of past pain. Others hold that the patient can block awareness to the current pain, or that the painful feeling can be substituted with a less noxious one, changing the patient's perception of the pain from negative to positive. As for pain associated with other ailments, The National Institutes of Health Assessment Panel on Integration of Behavioral and Relaxation Approaches reported in July 1996 that "strong evidence" existed for the ability of hypnosis to relieve pain associated with having cancer.

A patient must be very open to hypnosis for it to work because patients cannot be hypnotized against their will.

Imagery

Imagery is the practice of using the senses and the imagination to achieve an aim. It has gotten a lot of attention in the last twenty years, particularly in the sports world, where it has been used to improve performance. Hospitals are also employing it, sometimes with patients with cancer, to improve patients' ability to relax, to engage them in their own therapies, and to improve clinical outcome.

Typically, a therapist helps a patient relax and guides him through different situations that he imagines in his mind. The concept is that by imagining, say, a sports performance, rehearsing it mentally, and gaining confidence, the athlete will more likely succeed when the actual performance occurs. To engage the senses, a therapist might ask a basketball player, for example, to think of the smell of the ball or gym, a skier to imagine the sound of the skis on the snow, a football receiver to imagine the sound of the ball hitting his waiting hands. By concentrating on imagining the preferred outcome, patients get in touch, foremost, with what their most important aims are and, secondly, with those mental forces, conscious and unconscious, that are affecting their actions.

The patient who has chronic knee problems can visualize the knee as an asset instead of a liability. Imagery is also useful for cases requiring acute care. One psychotherapist who teaches imagery to cancer patients experienced a fracture of both leg bones near his ankle in a skiing accident. He used imagery to think positively of his bones healing, to focus on the disappearance of the fractures. He carried with him a trimmed photograph of a player running on a tennis court that showed only the healthy leg, and he imagined it as his own. It is the optimistic glass-is-half-full-not-half-empty approach. By not dwelling on the negative (disability or pain), the person moves on to the positive.

When I was team physician for the University of Missouri, I treated a basketball player who had injured his knee and was out for the season. When he returned the next year, he had problems with his confidence in shooting. A sports psychologist and the coaches worked with him. They preached to him a very common basketball philosophy, which was not to take a shot unless he was in his "spot" on the floor. This spot reflects the point on the court from which he achieved his best shooting. This therapy caused two things to happen: it increased his chances of making the shot and when he made it, it doubly increased his confidence in shooting from this spot and elsewhere. They had him imagine getting to his place on the court to take his "shot" and the ball going through the hoop.

It worked.

Laughter

Prescribing laughter as a therapy sounds silly, doesn't it? Well, that is just the point. The classic example of how laughter and the physiology that it evokes can cure illness is depicted in Norman Cousins's book *Anatomy of an Illness as Perceived by the Patient.* He points out that when he went through all of the traditional therapies he still had painful, disabling arthritis. He then proceeded to watch slapstick comedy and take in all the potential sources to evoke laughter and plain-old belly laughter that he could stand. Thereafter, he not only symptomatically felt better but he also saw a reduction in abnormal laboratory test values.

Dr. Steve Allen, Jr., son of the well-known television comedian, believes in the power of mirth and playfulness to transform the bumps in life's road into adventures instead of tests of survival. When not behind a desk as an academic administrator, he is often teaching audiences to juggle and preaching the creativity-building and health-enhancing power of laughter. When speaking to an audience in Houston once, he recounted his experiences of working as a physician briefly on a Zuni reservation in New Mexico. Integral to the Zuni hierarchy of healers, according to Allen, were not only medicine men and women but also two other "healers"—those who had survived a serious illness (who were considered to have special wisdom) and clowns (who were considered to be practitioners of a sacred art).

The Navajo also use a *heyoke,* or clown, as a healer. He dresses like a clown and does things backwards, riding his horse in ceremonies backwards and saying the opposite of what he means instead of speaking straightforwardly. This method of interacting pokes fun at empty form and is a two-edged sword—at once humorous and insightful.

Another who believes laughter is good medicine is Madan Kataria, the founder of Laughing Clubs International. One club's members, meeting outside a park in Bombay, India at 7 a.m. daily, chortled, giggled, and guffawed so loudly they prompted nearby residents to file a formal noise pollution complaint. Described in a *Health* magazine article by Mary Roach as "busting their guts for no apparent reason," Bombay's Jogger's Park Laughing Club rejected relying on jokes—eventually "silly" or "stale," Kataria says—and depends instead on exercises—"ho-ho, ha-ha, ho-ho, ha-ha"—to begin and the infectious quality of laughter to keep its members in the throes of hilarity. Some deep breathing and silent laughing (with mouth open) finish out the meeting. Some follow the laughing session with an exercise session. And this is only one of almost thirty clubs in the city.

The concept of laughter as medicine is at least as old as the Old Testament—"A merry heart doeth good like a medicine" (Proverbs 17:22)—but laughter's effects have been confirmed in small laboratory studies to stimulate the cerebral cortex, to serve as an aerobic equivalent to brief exercise, and to increase several measures of immune function. Not all studies impart health advantages to those who laugh, but, as Kataria points out, you don't have to worry about an overdose. The secret of its effect may have in part something to do with philosopher Thomas Hobbes's assertion that laughter gives those who laugh some eminence over others or over a less robust self they may have formerly been.

That assertion of good standing may have broader implications. It is confirmed by a survey showing that having a sense of humor can raise your ratings with your boss. Pennsylvania's Quaker Chemical Corporation in a 1993 review found that managers were more likely to rehire workers who had a sense of humor, who were well liked, and who worked well with others than they were workers who were only highly proficient.

Life has good and bad times, as does illness. Getting stuck on the negative, depressed side deters health; therefore, put on your white coat, wrap a stethoscope around your neck, and get your prescription pad. Do what Cousins did and what Allen and Kataria recommend. Write yourself a prescription for laughter.

Massage

The word *massage* comes from the Arabic word *massa,* meaning "to stroke," "to touch," or "to handle." Others have suggested it may have come from the Greek word *masso,* which means "to knead." Massage obviously can be done by anyone, but some practice massage after going to school and earning a massage license.

Therapeutic massage works to release muscle spasms and increase blood and lymph circulation. Of the two main types of massage, the gentle "feel good" type of massage, that has generally been termed *Swedish,* and Shiatsu, which was developed in Japan and described above (see Acupressure), Americans are more familiar with the former. Shiatsu is many times combined with other therapies.

In rhythmic, constant-contact Swedish massage there are four basic techniques: pressure, petrissage, percussion, effleurage. Pressure is exactly what you would think. It can be either longitudinal or circular motions and can vary from light tactile stimulation to deep pressure. Petrissage involves stretching muscles to relax them and deeper movement involving mobilization of the muscle, rolling it and grasping it. Percussion can be done by cupping the hands, hitting on the sides of the hands (hacking), clapping, or pummeling (with the fists). Effleurage is a constant rhythmic stroking of the hands always directing the push toward the heart.

Principal pain around a knee can be caused by tight muscles that attach to the knee; therefore, it is possible to have tight muscles in the back and tight hamstrings that result in tendonitis in the knee. Massaging solely around the knee would not relieve the pain because it would not fully relax the muscles in the chain.

I've had numerous patients with knee pain, specifically posterior knee pain, that were helped with massage. Very commonly, the massage and stretching needs to occur with the hamstring muscles, or muscles in the back of the leg, and also the low back. There is a chain, or continuum, of tightness from the low back to the hamstring muscles, and there can also be tightness in the calf muscles. This can all end up in pain in the back of the knee. Therefore, just massaging the back of the knee will not address the tightness in the other muscles.

In research with patients with cancer who are undergoing bone marrow transplantation, clinicians have tried massage to improve outcome. They found that patients who underwent complementary massage experienced less nausea and had lower blood pressure than those undergoing transplantation without it.

Meditation

Meditation essentially seeks a state of relaxation by focusing thoughts or projecting an image in the mind. It promotes clearing the mind through guided imagery, breathing exercises, or other technique. In one type of meditation, each individual uses a mantra, or repetitive incantation, to assist in achieving this state.

In a comparison study of transcendental meditation and progressive muscle relaxation in about one hundred inner city older African-Americans with mild to severe high blood pressure, both methods significantly reduced systolic and diastolic pressure but transcendental meditation's reductions were about twice those of progressive relaxation. The systolic pressure is the top number in the blood pressure fraction, and the diastolic pressure is the number on the bottom. In transcendental meditation, the individual seeks to achieve a state of being at rest but alert by repeating a mantra, a sound or phrase chanted or intoned like a repetitive prayer. In progressive muscle relaxation, the individual mentally moves from one anatomical muscle group to another, concentrating on relaxing each group until the body as a whole is relaxed. Though the changes were small, the decrease in risk of heart attack and stroke indicated by the fall in high blood pressure was important to these high-risk patients.

In another study of patients with documented coronary artery disease, 21 patients were assigned to a group using transcendental meditation or to a waiting list (no intervention). Both groups were pre-tested, and after eight months those who had used transcendental meditation had significantly lower heart rate and blood pressure values during exercise testing than did those who had undergone no treatment. They also had increases of more than 10 percent in exercise tolerance and in maximal workload capability.

Yoga exercises encompass meditation aspects to fully do the postures, thus achieving relaxation of the muscles. Meditation is very good for people who have chronic pain in their knee.

Music Therapy

Music therapy is a second-line assistant in managing pain. It in itself won't be enough, but it is a very good adjunct. Studies have shown that music can reduce postoperative pain, no matter what type of music or its volume. Its soothing influence has also been sought for the surgical suite. *Rolling Stone* labeled a physician on the first Texas heart transplant team "Rock Doc" for adding music for its soothing effect to the surgical experience. For the best effect in self-therapy, choose music you love, single out the stimulus (lie down, close your eyes, use headphones), and anticipate a beneficial, pain-relieving effect.

A "music" that has found its way onto compact discs and cassette tapes, increasing the pleasure of many, is the recording of sounds from nature. Birds singing, water falling, rivers rushing—these are sounds that delight and de-stress. Yes, it is better to be there yourself and to get the touch of the wind and the smell of the earth as well. But do not let your inability to go to the source prevent the source from coming to you. Practice responsive listening in listening to nature. Imagine what it is telling you. Try to recognize sound sources. Listen for patterns. Advocates of this kind of therapy tout its ability to relax and renew.

Neuromuscular Therapy

Neuromuscular therapy is a new name for an old technique, which is essentially deep pressure massage. The theory is that kneading and working the muscle very vigorously can decrease the spasm in the muscle. Sometimes this spasm isn't felt. It is more like an increased resting tension of the muscle; therefore, in dealing with tendonitises of the knee, such as patella tendonitis, a therapist could work on the quadriceps muscles all the way up to the hip. Many times within that muscle a specific area will be painful and quite tight. The treatments may initially cause more pain in the muscles before they totally relax and thus take the tension off another muscle and/or tendon. I have found neuromuscular therapy particularly helpful in hamstring problems going up to the knee.

Prayer

Turgenev said that "whatever a man prays for, he prays for a miracle. Every prayer reduces itself to this: 'Great God, grant that twice two be not four.'" In this basic sense, the spoken or unspoken petition to God or a god is a cry for help that will change reality. Parents often refer to their children as miracles. They are miracles because the parents have seen what the children have survived—childhood diseases; near misses with cars, trains, buses, and bikes; and other incidents only imaginable by parents who wait at home while children are away in the world on trips, at rock concerts, or in college. Other parents can boast of the miracle of a birth after years of infertility or the miracle of a child's recovery after a life-threatening illness. In those cases, "twice two" was not four.

Physician and author Larry Dossey calls prayer "tapping into the larger unfound self." Certainly in uttering the concerns closest to their hearts and in asking for strength and protection as they face them, those who pray are identifying and verbalizing the obstacles to peace in their own lives and may go on to imagine what must be done to resolve them. These are surely kindred to steps taken in psychotherapy. Others offer a more kinesthetic supplication by dancing their prayers. One dance studio offers two hours midday on Sundays for expression of prayers through dances of all kinds.

What happens in more traditional prayer sometimes is that what changes is not a situation but the person praying, who in turn changes the situation. In this sense, prayer is more than the direct request for divine intervention. It is an *experience* that changes, sometimes revolutionizes, the person praying. This is reflected in Shakespeare's *The Merchant of Venice:* "We do pray for mercy, / And that same prayer doth teach us all to render / The deeds of mercy."

Psychotherapy

There are over 250 different types of psychotherapy. Actually, there may be as many types as there are people's needs. Unquestionably, we all need some type of psychotherapy sometime, and we all get it from very different professional and nonprofessional sources. There are five main types of psychotherapy. **Psychodynamic therapy** is essentially psychoanalysis of the patient's past and how it affects the present. **Behavioral therapy** focuses on a change in behavior. **Cognitive therapy** examines the thoughts that underlie behavior. This therapy may be useful in mild depression. **Systems therapy** deals with relationship patterns. And **supportive therapy** is therapy used in an intense or acute emotional crisis. This helps the patient "get through it."

In a study at Northwest University Medical School, patients with hip fractures who underwent psychotherapy in the hospital went home sooner than those who did not undergo therapy. One of the main accomplishments of psychotherapy is encouraging patients to become mentally active and participatory in their healing. A condition called "reflex sympathetic dystrophy" in the knee has to do with weakness and pain in the knee with a psychological component. Psychotherapy in conjunction with physical therapy treatments is a mainstay for recovery.

Reflexology

Reflexology is a technique of digital pressure massage on the hands and feet with the belief that it will have a resultant effect on other areas of the body. Reflexologists manipulate specific points on the feet or hands to create an effect—improving circulation, reducing tension, stimulating healing—on a corresponding but distant part of the body. Developed in the East, reflexology is similar to acupuncture, but not all points can be equated to representative organ points in the feet. A reflexologist tries to diagnose abnormal pressure areas and free them up so that the corresponding organ will work better.

My only experience with this was with a patient who was having postoperative knee pain. He had gone to a reflexologist and learned specifically to push on the space between the first and second toe to decrease the pain in his knee. It relieved his pain and reduced his need for drugs.

Transcutaneous Neural Stimulation

Transcutaneous neural stimulation (TNS) is a method by which an electrical current is applied to the skin to decrease pain. Essentially electrical acupuncture, TNS is based on the theory that the pleasant stimulation from the TNS electrical paths or unit traverses the nerves quicker than the noxious stimuli through the pain nerves. Subsequently, this gets to the brain and, according to Melzak and Wall's gate theory, closes the gate to pain and the patient senses the good feeling. TNS has been used widely with relatively good results.

In the mid 1980s, some colleagues and I reported our results in using TNS postoperatively ("The Use of Transcutaneous Neural Stimulation and Isokinetic Testing in Arthroscopic Knee Surgery," *American Journal of Sports Medicine* 13:1, 1985). We found that not only was TNS useful in decreasing postoperative pain, but also it allowed patients to get their strength back quicker because they didn't hurt as much postoperatively. The article was published at a time when there was still considerable skepticism about TNS, and this research showed that it could work. Since then, others and I have used this technique a lot to decrease postoperative pain, particularly in lieu of using drugs or to decrease the amount of drugs a patient needs. TNS is excellent in treating chronic pain and preventing drug addiction that sometimes results with drug therapy. It can also be used in pregnancy when some drugs would be contraindicated. The electrical pads are placed on each side of the painful area. If the whole knee hurts, we put either two or four pads about the knee.

Yoga

Yoga is a program of exercises that when practiced can help one attain mental and physical control and a sense of well-being. An excellent combination of exercise and meditation, it can be used by anyone. Yoga builds strength, balance, and flexibility by gently stretching the spine, muscles, tendons, and joints. Again, this has been around for centuries. A common image Americans carry in their heads, probably from watching cartoons, is of a turban-topped yoga practitioner literally wrapped in a knot. In contrast to this contorted stereotype, yoga is excellent, with its slow stretches and resulting relaxation, for undoing the "knots" caused by stress. When yoga is practiced in a heated environment, such as Bikram Choudhury's Hot Yoga is, the body's resistance is relieved without risking injury, enabling you to stretch more deeply.

Patients to whom I have recommended yoga as therapy have had excellent results. An advantage is the class setting that affords the benefits and fun of being part of a group. Though, after one learns some of the maneuvers and stretches, they certainly can be done at home. Some postures can put too much stress on the knee ligaments, especially if they have been injured, so checking with a practitioner is the best prevention from further injury. A good teacher should not push you so hard that you experience pain the next day.

Conclusion

The array of complementary therapies presented here is just a hint of the broad range of therapies available. Many of these therapies require no special training and no special equipment; others require the expertise of a specialist. You, working with your physician, can find the best solution to your problem, but you will have to work together. As medical and scientific researchers examine the mechanisms of action, safety, and clinical effectiveness of these treatments, we will learn more about how to use them and the scope of their benefits and risks. You can make your own progress by talking to your doctor about what alternative and complementary therapies you use. I am sure that I am not the only physician who believes his patients rank among his best teachers.

8

Maintaining Balance

"Look to your health...value it next to a good conscience."
—Izaak Walton

Kim Zmeskal was a record-setter both on and off the gymnastics floor. In 1991, Zmeskal became the first American gymnast to win the all-around title at the World Championships. The next year, she was part of the bronze medal—winning team at the World Olympics in Barcelona. Also during this time, Zmeskal won the all-around title at the U.S. Nationals for three years straight. She went on to assist the U.S. Olympic Team, but when she was still a competitive gymnast, she faced a challenge to her success. She seriously injured her anterior cruciate ligament and had to undergo reconstructive surgery. In a dramatically brief recovery, she returned to gymnastics workouts in only four months after surgery. Many athletes take six to nine months to recover from this injury. In fact, some skiers who sustain this injury and undergo surgery do not return to sports until the following season. Recently, Super Bowl announcers commended some football players with this injury who returned to playing in about four months, highly praising them as if they were the only athletes to do it. When athletes like Zmeskal set a goal for recovery and achieve it, they do more than benefit themselves. They teach other athletes as well as their physicians important lessons in goal-setting. Most of us look at the highest standard and consider it the goal; they look at the highest standard and consider it a place to begin.

Our knees are an integral part of ourselves that we often take for granted, until they are affected by a twist, a blow, arthritis, or overuse. Injuries test our abilities to maintain our equilibrium, both literally and figuratively. Walking with the use of only one knee, not two, challenges us to physically balance as well as to feel confident. Being able to move without hindrance from one place to another is central to our concept of freedom and our concept of ourselves as capable men and women. Think of the athlete who is sidelined after a ligament injury, the middle-aged man who finds his knees less reliable during weekend chores and more likely to ache with overuse, and the elderly woman whose arthritis may force her to change her activities.

In part, because these challenges reshape our physical image, they have potential to reshape our psychological image of ourselves. Jung said that meaninglessness was equivalent to illness, and for some, the converse—that illness is equivalent to meaninglessness—is also true. Trying to bring our self-concept back to an upright position after an injury or loss of use may require as much attention and effort as bringing our physical being back into shape. The individual who suffers a heart attack, for example, may have to cope with depression as well as the new reality of his or her physical condition. Both physical and emotional adjustments must be made.

But this does not necessarily mean accepting whatever limitations others expect you to live within. The heroes of many a modern story are those who refused to accept the reality they were handed. Glenn Cunningham, the Kansan who in 1938 was first to run the indoor mile in four minutes (4:04.4), had first begun to exercise in a rehabilitation effort after his legs were severely burned in a schoolhouse fire. When the best record for the mile was 4:10 and it had been bettered on about 30 occasions, Cunningham was responsible for more than a third of the better records. Though as a child Wilma Rudolph fought polio, in Rome in 1960 she became the first American woman to win three gold medals in Olympic track and field events. Growing up in Tennessee, the African American woman faced paralysis that required bracing for support, but she went on to set world records in the 100-meter and 200-meter dashes, one before her Olympic victories and one after.

The 72—year—old grandmother who skis, the paraplegic who plays basketball aggressively from a wheelchair, the author who tirelessly submits a manuscript, rejection after rejection, and finally wins publication and praise—all refuse to be defined solely by what has happened to them and what others expect. It is this kind of thinking that can help you pull from injury a new life or can help you maintain balance you may have already achieved.

In these closing pages of the book, I want to review what we've talked about in terms of achieving a healthy lifestyle and overcoming injury. In this scenario, I am the physician writing a prescription; you are both patient and pharmacist because it will be your job to "fill" the prescriptions I write. Instead of a list of drugs, though, I am prescribing a list of initiatives for you to undertake. Just like undertaking exercises, you need to begin with a warm-up period. By that I mean that you should institute changes gradually. Do not require too much of yourself all at once. Everyone has his or her own speed at which to work. Expect the change to make a difference. Think creatively about how life will improve with these changes. These "prescriptions" include recommendations for emotional as well as physical revitalization.

1. **Control your weight**. What would you give to live a long life? If you could rub a magic lamp and have the secret of a long life revealed to you, would you perform the task without hesitating? Well, if you rub the lamp of scientific study, the revelation that will come to you is that to have a long life you must control your weight. More than any other factor, maintaining a healthy body weight is central to longevity. If you are able to maintain a healthy body weight, you will be bucking a trend. Since 1960, the number of obese Americans has increased by about a third to 61 million.

Gaining weight and decreasing activity becomes a vicious cycle that eventually incorporates a stiffness that discourages the activity your body needs and encourages the weight gain that will ensure the cycle's continuation. If you maintain a healthy body weight, your knees will have an easier time supporting you and you will be taking a major step toward preventing degenerative joint disease. In addition, you will be improving your cardiovascular health—reducing your risk of high blood pressure, diabetes, high cholesterol, and, depending on what you eat and don't eat, some cancers.

Furthermore, you will be setting a good example for the children in your family. Children and adolescents are not immune to the trend toward obesity in America. Between 1963 and 1994, the proportion of overweight children and adolescents in the United States had risen from 4 percent to 11 percent, according to the National Health and Nutrition Examination Survey. This increase, according to the federal government, poses a substantial barrier to achieving overall health goals in the new millennium's first decade.

To control your weight, follow the recommendations for good nutrition in this book or follow the American Heart Association's heart-healthy diet recommendations. Like quitting smoking, controlling your weight is something you must do for yourself, something for which you must take personal responsibility. Don't be discouraged if you start to overeat again. Just start over. Take it one day at a time, and control negative thoughts that can undermine your efforts.

2. **Exercise regularly**. The benefits of exercising regularly are difficult to overestimate. Regular exercise is fundamental to preventing knee injuries, it familiarizes the joint with movement, and it increases your awareness of what your body can or cannot do. Exercising can strengthen muscles, increase flexibility, and improve endurance. Tendons and ligaments are likely to benefit, too. Like the body check described in Chapter 2, exercising puts you in touch with your body and its limitations.

I like to emphasize that our bodies are "hard-wired" for exercise. Throughout time, until the very recent past, human beings had to use their bodies to keep their bodies—they had to work hard to make sure food was available. Without physical effort on their part—hunting and foraging formerly and physical labor until recently—human beings could not sustain life. Evolutionary changes haven't caught up with the industrial and technological advances that now require fewer and fewer of us in Western civilization to rely on our brawn. Our bodies are made to be used, to be stretched, exercised, and challenged. Without exercise, our bodies grow less and less able to perform even necessary everyday tasks.

A sedentary lifestyle can be costly. Recent estimates of the risk of physical inactivity attributed to it about a third of coronary heart disease, a third of colon cancer, and a third of diabetes cases diagnosed in adults. Dr. Steven Blair of the Cooper Institute for Aerobics Research in Dallas and his colleagues found that low physical fitness was associated with higher chance of death, no matter whether those compared were smokers or not or whether cholesterol level or blood pressure was high. "Low fitness is an important precursor of mortality," the report stated in its conclusion. Furthermore, low physical fitness over decades of life leads to functional limitations in old age; in fact, a national health survey found that 38 percent of Americans 65 years of age and older had at least one functional limitation.

The good news is that changes from a sedentary lifestyle to an active lifestyle have been associated with falling death rates similar to those seen in smokers who quit smoking. And it is never too late to improve; one researcher found that muscular strength can be doubled by resistance training even into the tenth decade of life. One system of exercises recommended for older Americans to improve balance, muscular strength, and aerobic power, thereby minimizing the threat of functional limitation, is T'ai Chi. This ancient Chinese discipline employs contemplative movements in an organized way and can be implemented in community settings without high technology or highly trained individuals, thereby increasing its practicality. For older individuals in particular, it is important to note that T'ai Chi training appears to reduce the risk of multiple falls.

But how much physical activity is enough? In a report that aimed to answer this question, a workshop spun off from the group that wrote the American Heart Association's Medical/Scientific Statement on Exercise in 1992 said that neither the minimal nor the maximal amounts of exercise for benefit are known. But one thing is certain: "The evidence is clear," the workshop participants wrote, "that high intensity is not necessary to appreciably reduce the risk of coronary heart disease." The report pointed out that moderately intense activities carry less risk than vigorous activities of orthopedic injury and such cardiovascular events as heart attacks. This should not be misinterpreted to mean that *maximal* benefit can be gained from *moderate* effort. What is important is that you do something sometime. Options in selecting activities and in parceling them into multiple shorter experiences, accumulated over a day—an improvement over traditional single-session exercise programs—are changes that may encourage more people to become physically active.

Consistency is more important than intensity. A swim at the local pool. A bike ride. A walk. Even five minutes is better than no time at all. If exercising seems impossible to fit into your schedule, it may be because you insist on pursuing an ideal program. Your work or family schedule may not permit you to go to a health club or join an exercise class. You may need to set up a second-hand exercise bike by your phone, the television, or the table where your children do their homework. You may need to walk to a nearby retailer rather than drive. Perhaps you could persuade the buddy you lunch with to walk or run with you during part of your noontime break. You may want to engage your family in a trip to a park rather than a trip to the mall. Don't be intimidated by advertising's promotion of the "right" thing to wear or the "right" activity. Your muscles and tendons won't know what you have on.

3. **Get the mental and physical rest you need**. Take time to relax and make sure you are getting enough sleep. Sleep requirements vary among individuals, and because we do not do the same thing every day, our levels of need change daily. Age also is a major factor in determining how much sleep we need. If you are having trouble getting out of bed in the morning, if you feel overly drowsy during the day, and if you rely on coffee, caffeine-containing soft drinks, or pills to keep you awake, you do not need an expert to tell you that you need more sleep. One

especially stressed writer I knew told me that during one grant-writing marathon she was so tired that the brief quiet at a stop light was enough to make her fall asleep.

Without sleep, we are not our best selves. We may be grumpy. We may have fatigue that diminishes our defenses against infection. The accuracy and speed with which we perform physical and mental tasks may be impaired, as may our judgment. Without proper rest, tired muscle does not have time to repair, rebuild, or to restore its energy.

What sleep you lose during the week, you should try and make up on the weekends. Sleep in when you can. Take a "power nap" in the early afternoon. Certain cultures incorporate time for a midday nap into their schedules. If sleeplessness has more to do with chronic anxiety and lying awake in bed at night rather than scheduling, you may want to consult a psychologist, therapist, or medical sleep clinic about what is keeping you awake.

4. **Reduce stress**. In an unexplained paradox, Americans have more leisure time than they did in the 1960s, but they continue to feel the pinch of time. Thirty eight percent of Americans reported feeling rushed in a 1992 survey conducted by scholars. In the National Health Interview Surveys, more than half of those interviewed (56 percent) reported "a lot" or "moderate" stress within the last two weeks of the interview. Women are more likely to be stressed than men, and people who are 35 to 44 years of age are more likely to be stressed than those in other age groups. More money and more education translate into more stress. Scholars John P. Robinson and Geoffrey Godbey, whose surveys unearthed some of these findings, theorize that people feel more rushed now because they are always trying to do more, a behavior they call *time-deepening*. They see people using four tactics to get more out of the time they have: trying to speed up an activity; substituting a shorter activity for a longer one; multitasking, or doing more than one activity at a time; and approaching activities with greater time consciousness.

But things may be changing. With a follow-up study in 1995, the proportion of interviewees saying they felt stressed fell to 34 percent, and the percentage saying they felt like they had less time than in the past fell from a majority to a minority (from 54 percent to 45 percent). In an ironic twist, the activity that Americans say they are most willing to give up—television watching—is the activity to which they devote most of their spare time—21 hours per week. But researchers Robinson and Godbey remind us that many viewers, especially women, perform household tasks while watching television, and turning it off would not turn all those hours into "spare" time.

Stress wears on us like a stress fracture on a bone. Usually the result of overuse, stress fractures are hairline cracks that appear in bones and that will progress to a full break if rest isn't allowed to restore the bone. Both the thigh (fibula) and shin (tibia) bones may suffer fractures, but they are more common in the tibia. Stress wears on our spirits, just as these fractures threaten the bones.

Though perceptions of the meaning and scope of stresses vary, the response is typically adaptation. If the adaptation is successful, equilibrium will be restored; if the adaptation is not, coping may stretch into a long process. Stress is often caused by loss—a death, divorce, a promotion or job loss, or physical injury. This loss and the resultant frustration can be compounded by a loss of drive or ambition, caused by the depression connected to the first loss.

To prevent a downward spiral, we must respond. Two common forms of adaptation are problem solving and conscious relaxation. These are not the only adaptations that can be made; they are simply two that many people use to combat stress. They may be used singly or in combination. In problem solving, the problem causing the stress is evaluated, a plan made, and its implementation evaluated. Steps are often outlined as follows:

- Define the problem and identify the problem's cause.
- Acknowledge any personal behavior that may contribute to the problem, and brainstorm solutions.
- Evaluate each solution, and select one to try.
- Put plan into action.
- After a predetermined time, reevaluate the solution, and modify or replace as necessary.

Another way to deal with stress is to practice meditation with conscious relaxation. The following method, described by Dr. Harold Jensen of Harvard, can be practiced once or twice a day in any quiet place and requires no specific change in lifestyle except the time commitment to perform the meditation. Do not practice this meditation within two hours after eating a meal, so that the body is not lethargic and is relaxed rather than focused on digestion.

1. Sit quietly in a comfortable position.
2. Close your eyes.
3. Begin the process of relaxing your muscles. You will begin at

your feet and move up. Consciously relax your muscles as you move up your body.

4. Breathe consciously. Close your mouth and breathe through your nose. Pay attention to your breathing, saying "one" silently to yourself as you exhale and repeating it as you inhale. The aim in repeating this word is to focus on the meditation and to drive away distracting thoughts.

5. Practice this conscious relaxation for twenty minutes. Add to this time a few minutes to sit quietly before resuming your everyday life. Do not use an alarm to end your meditation. Simply open your eyes to check the time.

6. Do not measure your performance. Simply remain passive and let relaxation occur. With practice, relaxation should come easily.

One of the benefits of practicing this procedure is that it provides the mental rest mentioned earlier.

5. **Build a partnership with the physicians and other health care professionals you consult.** As I have tried to emphasize in these pages, the responsibility for the health of an individual is shared by both doctor and patient. Working together as a team, they can experience a give-and-take that brings added dimension to the physician-patient relationship. That relationship ideally should be characterized by openness, respect, warmth, and empathy.

Choosing a doctor who shares your philosophy of the patient-physician relationship and who is qualified to treat your ailment can be a challenge. If you are choosing someone to treat your knee problem, you need an orthopedist who is board certified. To verify certification, you can visit the American Board of Medical Specialties at *http://www. abms.org* and, after successfully logging on, click Who's Certified? The board issues consumers passwords after they register.

Fighting the Fractures of Modern Life

Your knees were millions of years in the making and were formed in your mother's womb in little more than a month. That the knee is the most complex joint in the human body is not surprising. What is surprising is the longevity of its simple design, its quick embryonic development, and how well it functions for a lifetime with little maintenance. The miracle of the knee's operation—the ability to carry massive weight compounded by movement, to twist while bearing weight, to carry the ball all the way to the goal line or basket, to function divinely despite the absence of a mechanical interface—is what makes the knee so remarkable. Often overlooked, frequently disdained, our knees remind us simultaneously of our strength and our weakness, our ability to walk upright and the possibility of being bent-kneed in submission.

Maintain balance in your life. Get enough rest. Fight the fractures in your life that stress would induce. Take time to problem solve or find calm through conscious relaxation. Assume responsibility for your health in partnership with your physician, and walk tall, knowing all that implies.